AF194382

Poultry Inspection

The Basis for a Risk-Assessment Approach

Prepared by the
Committee on Public Health Risk Assessment of Poultry Inspection Programs
Food and Nutrition Board
Commission on Life Sciences
National Research Council

National Academy Press
Washington, D.C. 1987

NOTICE: The project that is the subject of this report was approved by the Governing Board of the National Research Council, whose members are drawn from the councils of the National Academy of Sciences, the National Academy of Engineering, and the Institute of Medicine. The members of the committee responsible for the report were chosen for their special competences and with regard for appropriate balance. This report has been reviewed by a group other than the authors according to procedures approved by a Report Review Committee consisting of members of the National Academy of Sciences, the National Academy of Engineering, and the Institute of Medicine.

The National Academy of Sciences is a private, nonprofit, self-perpetuating society of distinguished scholars engaged in scientific and engineering research, dedicated to the furtherance of science and technology and to their use for the general welfare. Upon the authority of the charter granted to it by the Congress in 1863, the Academy has a mandate that requires it to advise the federal government on scientific and technical matters. Dr. Frank Press is president of the National Academy of Sciences.

The National Academy of Engineering was established in 1964, under the charter of the National Academy of Sciences, as a parallel organization of outstanding engineers. It is autonomous in its administration and in the selection of its members, sharing with the National Academy of Sciences the responsibility for advising the federal government. The National Academy of Engineering also sponsors engineering programs aimed at meeting national needs, encourages education and research, and recognizes the superior achievements of engineers. Dr. Robert M. White is president of the National Academy of Engineering.

The Institute of Medicine was established in 1970 by the National Academy of Sciences to secure the services of eminent members of appropriate professions in the examination of policy matters pertaining to the health of the public. The Institute acts under the responsibility given to the National Academy of Sciences by its congressional charter to be an adviser to the federal government and, upon its own initiative, to identify issues of medical care, research, and education. Dr. Samuel O. Thier is president of the Institute of Medicine.

The National Research Council was organized by the National Academy of Sciences in 1916 to associate the broad community of science and technology with the Academy's purposes of furthering knowledge and advising the federal government. Functioning in accordance with general policies determined by the Academy, the Council has become the principal operating agency of both the National Academy of Sciences and the National Academy of Engineering in providing services to the government, the public, and the scientific and engineering communities. The Council is administered jointly by both Academies and the Institute of Medicine. Dr. Frank Press and Dr. Robert M. White are chairman and vice chairman, respectively, of the National Research Council.

The study summarized in this report was supported by the Food Safety and Inspection Service of the U.S. Department of Agriculture under Contract No. 53-3A94-4-01.

LIBRARY OF CONGRESS CATALOG CARD NUMBER 87-60910
INTERNATIONAL STANDARD BOOK NUMBER 0-309-03743-3

Printed in the United States of America
First Printing, May 1987
Second Printing, July 1987

iii

COMMITTEE ON PUBLIC HEALTH RISK ASSESSMENT OF POULTRY INSPECTION PROGRAMS

JOSEPH RODRICKS (Chairman), Environ Corp., Washington, D.C.

JOHN C. BAILAR III (Vice Chairman), Harvard School of Public Health, Harvard University, Boston, Mass., and Office of Disease Prevention and Health Promotion, U.S. Department of Health and Human Services, Washington, D.C.

THOMAS GRUMBLY, Health Effects Institute, Cambridge, Mass.

MILEY W. MERKHOFER, Applied Decision Analysis, Inc., Menlo Park, Calif.

J. GLENN MORRIS, School of Medicine, University of Maryland, Baltimore, Md.

MORRIS POTTER, Division of Bacterial Diseases, Centers for Disease Control, U.S. Public Health Service, Atlanta, Ga.

MICHAEL PULLEN, Department of Large Animal Clinical Sciences, College of Veterinary Medicine, University of Minnesota, St. Paul, Minn.

National Research Council Staff

ROBERT A. MATHEWS, Project Manager

SHAKUNTALA CHAUBE, Program Officer

FARID E. AHMED, Senior Program Officer

FRANCES PETER, Editor

ELIZABETH J. HAMILL, Research Assistant

KAMAR PATEL, Secretary

SUSHMA PALMER, Director, Food and Nutrition Board

FOOD AND NUTRITION BOARD

KURT J. ISSLEBACHER (<u>Chairman</u>), Department of Gastroenterology, Massachusetts General Hospital, Boston, Mass.

RICHARD J. HAVEL (<u>Vice Chairman</u>), Cardiovascular Research Institute, University of California School of Medicine, San Francisco, Calif.

HAMISH N. MUNRO (<u>Vice Chairman</u>), USDA Human Nutrition Research Center on Aging, Tufts University, Boston, Mass.

WILLIAM E. CONNOR, Department of Medicine, Oregon Health Sciences University, Portland, Oreg.

PETER GREENWALD, Division of Cancer Prevention and Control, National Cancer Institute, Bethesda, Md.

M. R. C. GREENWOOD, Department of Biology, Vassar College, Poughkeepsie, N.Y.

JOAN D. GUSSOW, Department of Nutrition Education, Teachers College, Columbia University, New York, N.Y.

JAMES R. KIRK, Research and Development, Campbell Soup Company, Camden, N.J.

BERNARD J. LISKA, Department of Food Science, Purdue University, West Lafayette, Ind.

REYNALDO MARTORELL, Food Research Institute, Stanford University, Stanford, Calif.

WALTER MERTZ, Human Nutrition Research Center, Agricultural Research Service, U.S. Department of Agriculture, Beltsville, Md.

MALDEN C. NESHEIM, Division of Nutritional Sciences, Cornell University, Ithaca, N.Y.

RONALD C. SHANK, Department of Community and Environmental Medicine and Department of Pharmacology, University of California, Irvine, Calif.

ROBERT H. WASSERMAN, Department/Section of Physiology, New York State College of Veterinary Medicine, Ithaca, N.Y.

MYRON WINICK, Institute of Human Nutrition, College of Physicians and Surgeons, Columbia University, New York, N.Y.

J. MICHAEL McGINNIS (<u>Ex Officio</u>), Office of Disease Prevention and Health Promotion, Department of Health and Human Services, Washington, D.C.

ARNO G. MOTULSKY (<u>Ex Officio</u>), Center for Inherited Diseases, University of Washington, Seattle, Wash.

National Research Council Staff

SUSHMA PALMER, Director

Preface

In 1985, a committee of the National Research Council's Food and Nutrition Board (FNB) completed a report on the scientific basis of the Department of Agriculture's (USDA) meat and poultry inspection programs. In that study, at the request of the Food Safety and Inspection Service (FSIS) the committee specifically considered whether bird-by-bird inspection as currently done should be modified to a less-than-continuous procedure. The committee concluded that before the traditional postmortem inspection methods are displaced, a comparative risk analysis of traditional and modified inspection procedures is needed. In other words, FSIS should first determine the relative effectiveness of the inspection procedures that would replace the traditional methods. In response to this observation, the FSIS Administrator requested that the National Research Council conduct a follow-up study, specifically regarding poultry production, with the following objectives:

- Development of a risk-assessment model applicable to the poultry production system and an explanation of how it might be used to evaluate poultry inspection procedures.
- A general evaluation of current FSIS poultry inspection programs using the conceptual framework of the model.
- An assessment of the advantages of incorporating statistical sampling into poultry inspection procedures.

In response, a committee was appointed to conduct the study under the auspices of FNB within the Commission on Life Sciences. The multidisciplinary group appointed contained members with expertise in public health, food microbiology, toxicology, risk assessment, risk management, veterinary pathology, poultry inspection technology, biostatistics, and epidemiology. In cooperation with FSIS a formal charge was developed to guide the committee's work.

The information used to prepare this report included data from FSIS, the scientific literature, and other sources. The committee also had the opportunity to visit and inspect two poultry production plants. Opinions regarding the usefulness of poultry inspection were heard from federal veterinarians, poultry producers, and consumer representatives. The committee met five times during the study to review and evaluate this information with the goal of producing a report with conclusions and recommendations that would be useful to FSIS.

A summary of the committee's findings, conclusions, and recommendations appears in Chapter 1, The Executive Summary. Chapter 2 provides a historical background and a description of current poultry procedures. In Chapter 3 the committee describes its risk model. Chapters 4 and 5 apply the model to identify risks associated with microbiological and chemical contamination of poultry. The current FSIS poultry inspection program is evaluated in Chapter 6. Chapter 7 is a review of the conclusions and recommendations of the committee.

The committee expresses its appreciation to the following USDA staff members who were instrumental in arranging the site visit and providing information about poultry inspection procedures: Douglas Berndt, Robert Cook, William James, Marshall McCoulskey, Judith Segal, and John Prucha.

The committee is grateful for the invaluable assistance of the following people who provided testimony or written material: Diane Heiman, Public Voice for Food and Health Policy; Edward Mennings, National Association of Federal Veterinarians; Carl Telleen, National Joint Council for Food Inspection Locals; and Frank Craig, National Broiler Council. The committee is also grateful to Frederick A. Murphy, Leigh A. Sawyer, and Jeffrey A. Farrar of the Division of Viral Diseases, Center for Infectious Diseases, Centers for Disease Control, who provided information on avian vital diseases.

On behalf of the committee I would also like to thank Zain Abedin, Farid Ahmed, Shakuntala Chaube, and Robert Mathews of the FNB staff for providing the organizational and administrative support needed to complete the report in a timely manner. We wish also to acknowledge the contributions of Sushma Palmer, Director of FNB, and the assistance of Frances Peter, CLS editor; Elizabeth Hamill, FNB research assistant; and Kamar Patel, project secretary.

Of course, the report could not have been completed without the unfailing volunteer efforts of the committee. I am grateful for their commitment to preparing a document of the highest quality.

JOSEPH RODRICKS

CHAIRMAN

COMMITTEE ON PUBLIC HEALTH RISK ASSESSMENT OF POULTRY INSPECTION PROGRAMS

Contents

Chapter 1

Executive Summary

The production, slaughter, and distribution of broiler chickens (fryers) has become a major food industry that touches the lives of most Americans. Poultry products are currently consumed at a rate of well over 4 billion birds per year in the United States. Those products that pass through the inspection system required by law are, for the most part, wholesome. But because these products are potentially important vehicles of bacterial and chemical contaminants, the primary government agency charged with the oversight of poultry slaughter, the Food Safety and Inspection Service (FSIS) of the U.S. Department of Agriculture (USDA), has for the past decade been attempting to improve the effectiveness of poultry inspection by studying, testing, and reviewing several modifications of the existing program. Its goal has been to develop a system that retains the bird-by-bird inspection mandated by law, incorporates new technological advances, and more directly addresses public health concerns.

In 1983, recognizing the need to evaluate these proposed changes in inspection procedures, the Administrator of FSIS requested that the Food and Nutrition Board (FNB) of the National Research Council (NRC) examine the scientific basis of USDA's meat and poultry inspection program. The committee appointed to perform that task, the Committee on the Scientific Basis of the Nation's Meat and Poultry Inspection Programs, thoroughly evaluated current FSIS inspection programs. During the course of its study of those programs the committee observed that it could not find a comprehensive statement of criteria justifying inspection procedures, a systematic data base on contaminants, or a technically complete analysis of the benefits to human health resulting from the inspection process. That is, in general it found that it is not possible to determine from existing data whether current inspection programs actually fulfill their goal of protecting the public health. That committee considered whether to recommend a move to one of the newly proposed, less-than-continuous postmortem inspection systems but concluded that no such changes should be recommended until justified by a detailed risk analysis of the public health risks involved. It recommended that FSIS establish a risk-assessment program and apply formal risk-assessment procedures to assist in planning and evaluating all phases of poultry production in which hazards to public health might occur.

In response to that committee's assessment, which was published in 1985,[1] FSIS requested that FNB conduct another study to develop a risk-assessment model for comparing the effects on public health that might result from different postmortem inspection goals and strategies, to evaluate the public health risks associated with broiler chickens, and to review the advantages of a sampling program as part of an overall quality assurance program for poultry slaughter.

This report describes the findings of the Committee on Public Health Risk Assessment of USDA Poultry Inspection Programs, which was appointed to conduct the second study. The committee began its task by reviewing the ways in which traditional and new inspection procedures are related to public health. It soon decided that to evaluate poultry-related public health risks properly, it would be necessary to consider in addition to postmortem inspection various aspects of the poultry processing system outside the purview of FSIS, for example, growing conditions, preparation and handling, and cooking. Viewing the poultry processing system as a whole, the committee developed a conceptual risk-assessment model that could serve as a prototype for assessing public health risks associated with the entire spectrum of activities involved in poultry production, slaughter, processing, preparation, and consumption (referred to in this summary as the poultry system). It then evaluated the two most important health hazards associated with poultry—microbial and chemical contaminants —within the context of the model.

The conclusions and recommendations described in the following paragraphs derive from the committee's qualitative application of the model to the available information on poultry health hazards. Since the current data base is essentially the same as that used in the 1985 report, the present committee did not conduct another comprehensive evaluation of the FSIS poultry inspection program but, rather, focused on developing the risk-assessment model and delineating how it might be used to evaluate FSIS programs. As requested by FSIS, emphasis in this report has been placed on the use of risk assessment as a tool for evaluation. Some aspects of risk management that may lead to solutions of risk problems by FSIS are briefly described in Chapters 3, 4, and 5.

GENERAL CONCLUSIONS

The committee concluded that a risk-assessment approach is needed to evaluate health hazards associated with poultry. Accordingly, it developed a risk model, which is divided into submodels representing five different phases of the poultry system. These submodels are

---

[1] The committee's report, <u>Meat and Poultry Inspection</u>: <u>The Scientific Basis of the Nation's Program</u>, was published by the National Academy Press.

further broken down into various components. The model can be used to identify sources of health hazards, to suggest means of controlling their introduction, and to assess uncertainties in the ability to link public health consequences with specific hazards. Because the structure of any model reflects the particular perspective and knowledge of its designers, the conclusions and recommendations of the committee based on its model reflect its perception of how the poultry industry is most logically and usefully subdivided.

As stated in Chapter 3, the committee concluded that the present system of continuous inspection provides little opportunity to detect or control the most significant health risks associated with broiler chickens. Although information is not sufficient for the committee to conclude that the FSIS inspection program has no public health benefits, the weight of the evidence does suggest that the current program can not provide effective protection against the risks presented by microbial agents that are pathogenic to humans.

The committee concluded that risk assessment is one of the most valuable tools available to serve regulatory agencies such as FSIS because it facilitates a structured approach to the evaluation of information as well as an explicit, consistent, and logical treatment of data. Furthermore, it heightens awareness of uncertainties in the data and entails consideration of current scientific knowledge. If risk assessment were to be used by FSIS to identify health hazards associated with poultry, the most likely outcome would be to reduce public exposure to those hazards. This outcome would be dependent on implementing procedures that assign priorities based on the potential for reducing the magnitude of risk associated with a given hazard and on the prevention of risks instead of coping with them after they are present.

An effective risk-management program will consist of several monitoring activities, some of which are outside FSIS authority. Therefore, a comprehensive effort to protect the public from poultry-associated hazards will require an active and consistent liaison between FSIS and other government agencies. Attempts to control these public health risks could be significantly compromised without such interagency cooperation.

The committee confirmed that the current data base can serve as the basis for a comprehensive, quantitative risk assessment only for certain well-characterized chemical residues. For many purposes, however, including initial planning and evaluation of inspection strategies, it is sufficient and useful to perform qualitative assessments, such as that done by the committee in this report.

GENERAL RECOMMENDATIONS

- FSIS should adopt the well-established precepts of risk assessment as an integral part of its strategy to identify and manage public health risks associated with poultry. The committee's risk model can serve as a prototype that FSIS can refine by applying its extensive knowledge of the poultry system.

- FSIS should evaluate the current inspection system by using the risk-assessment model proposed by the committee and on the basis of its findings, modify the system so that it more directly addresses public health concerns.
- Rather than focusing on one procedure, such as bird-by-bird inspection, as the primary component of an inspection process, FSIS should direct its efforts toward the establishment of a comprehensive quality assurance program. Such a program would consist of several components, one of which might be organoleptic inspection.
- Emphasis should be shifted from detection to prevention of problems at the earliest feasible stage in production to increase the effectiveness of poultry risk-management activities.

A RISK-ASSESSMENT MODEL FOR POULTRY-ASSOCIATED HAZARDS

The process of risk assessment requires first a conceptual framework and second a risk model. For its conceptual framework, the committee adopted the well-accepted view of the role and nature of risk assessment developed in 1983 by the National Research Council's Committee on the Institutional Means for Assessment of Risks to Public Health, which proposed that risk assessment proceed in four steps: hazard identification, dose-response assessment, exposure assessment, and risk characterization. The use of these four steps helps to ensure the inclusion of all factors that determine risk. Successful execution of the final step, risk characterization, is dependent on the development and application of a model such as that proposed by the committee in Chapter 3.

In developing its model, the committee reviewed the major risk agents (pathogenic microorganisms or their toxins, and chemical residues) associated with the five major divisions (or submodels) of the poultry system: production (grow-out); slaughter; packing and processing; distribution and preparation; and consumption. The model includes all phases of processing in which hazards might be present, the sources from which risk agents are generated or released, routes of human exposure, and mechanisms by which the exposure can result in adverse health effects. The model provides one possible approach to the evaluation of current FSIS inspection programs. It can serve as a guide in the development of future programs and assist in determining the level of public health protection afforded by current inspection procedures.

Conclusions

- The committee concluded that by conducting a qualitative examination of each component of the risk model it is possible to identify potential sources of health hazards and to suggest means of preventing their introduction.

- The committee's assessment suggests that to minimize public health risks, the traditional focus on slaughter should be expanded to include other potential sources of poultry-related hazards, such as production, preparation and handling, and cooking.
- Although qualitative risk assessments, such as those undertaken by the committee, are often sufficient to identify hazards and their probable sources, quantitative assessments are required to establish the validity and mechanisms of cause-and-effect relationships and to identify the magnitude of public health problems.
- As FSIS evaluates the poultry processing system with the objective of increasing public health protection, its managerial personnel will have to identify those circumstances in which quantitative assessments are justified on the basis of additional insights or improved clarity that they could lend to the decision-making process.

Recommendations

- The committee's risk model should be regarded as a prototype that FSIS can modify and refine to suit its own special needs and goals.
- FSIS should attempt to ensure that all aspects of the poultry system are included in any risk model used, even if certain areas fall within the purview of other agencies.
- Qualitative risk assessments should form the initial bases for planning and selecting inspection and quality assurance programs. Quantitative assessments should be used when qualitative assessments prove inadequate and when sufficient data are available.

MICROBIOLOGICAL HAZARDS AND POULTRY

Salmonella species and Campylobacter jejuni from all sources (i.e., not from chickens alone) are each responsible for up to 2,000 cases of gastroenteric disease per 100,000 people per year in the United States. Illnesses caused by these microorganisms tend to be most severe among the very young, the very old, or patients with immunosuppressive diseases. The rate of infection tends to increase with increasing size of the inoculum (dose), although a relatively low inoculum is sometimes capable of causing disease in humans. The potential for introduction of Salmonella and Campylobacter, the most commonly encountered human pathogens on chicken, is highly variable and may occur at multiple points during production, slaughter, and processing. After reviewing data related to the occurrence, potential for causing infection, and pathogenicity for humans of several microbial species known to be present on chicken, the committee drew the following conclusions, which are described in greater detail in Chapter 4.

Conclusions

- Current inspection programs are not designed to detect the most important human pathogens found on poultry. This is evident from the reviews of FSIS inspection programs conducted by the present committee and the earlier Committee on the Scientific Basis of the Nation's Meat and Poultry Inspection Program.
- Minimizing microbial contaminants on poultry is a worthwhile objective, but it is premature to establish formal microbiological criteria for classifying raw products as microbiologically acceptable or unacceptable. The committee concluded that the data required to justify such formal regulatory standards do not exist..
- There is conclusive evidence that microorganisms pathogenic to humans (such as Salmonella and Campylobacter) are present on poultry at the time of slaughter and at retail.
- There is evidence linking disease in humans to the presence of pathogens on chickens. For example, epidemiological studies indicate that approximately 48% of Campylobacter infections are attributable to chicken. Data also suggest that chicken is probably an important source of salmonellosis in the United States.
- It is not known with certainty whether bacteria, viruses, and parasites that are common causes of disease in poultry can serve as food-borne pathogens for humans. Most of these organisms do not appear to be pathogenic in humans, but some may be. Thus, more data on the pathogenicity of these organisms are needed.

Recommendations

The association between microorganisms in and on poultry at slaughter and the occurrence of disease in humans is complex. Several potential sources of contamination exist throughout the poultry system. The committee recognizes, therefore, that attempts to resolve this problem will be correspondingly difficult and may require collaboration with other agencies. On the basis of its review of the literature and established principles of microbiology, however, the committee recommends that certain actions such as the following be taken to reduce the potential for disease to be caused by poultry-borne microorganisms.

- The ongoing search for data on microbial risks should continue and be complemented by new research. Emphasis should be placed on the prevention of human disease rather than on simple control of microbial counts during slaughter and processing.
- Potentially pathogenic microorganisms on poultry should be identified, the potential for exposure to an infectious dose of each pathogen should be determined, and the potential impact on public health that would result from the failure to control exposures should be evaluated.
- The critical control points at which known pathogenic microorganisms such as Salmonella and Campylobacter may be introduced into the poultry system should be identified and monitored, preferably

as a part of an HACCP (Hazard Analysis Critical Control Point) program.

- A population-based surveillance program should be established so that disease occurrence can be correlated with inspection strategies. This will require measuring the level of pathogenic microorganisms on market-ready poultry as well as establishing a system for surveillance of disease within a well-defined population.

- A range of educational programs for people who raise poultry and for those who handle raw broilers in slaughterhouses, at retail, and during food preparation in the home and commercial establishments should be developed or intensified. As part of this effort, poultry products should be labeled at retail to inform consumers how to handle the poultry to prevent diseases originating from microbial contaminants.

CHEMICAL HAZARDS AND POULTRY

The 1985 report <u>Meat and Poultry Inspection</u> contained a description and evaluation of the National Residue Program (NRP), which is the only formal program for monitoring chemical contaminants in poultry. In that report the committee concluded that the fundamental design of NRP needs to be improved to ensure protection from chemical hazards. In particular, it questioned the adequacy of sampling sizes and procedures, the basis for and the utility of tolerance levels as currently set, and the basis for setting priorities for testing. In light of these conclusions, the present committee approached its analysis of chemical risks by reviewing the current status of toxicological testing used in chemical risk assessments, by describing where information and data are needed to appropriately characterize various classes of chemicals, and by delineating eight necessary components of a program for controlling chemical contaminants (see Chapter 5). After examining data on the identification, toxicological properties, and occurrence of chemical hazards in poultry, and considering this information in the context of its model, the committee reached the conclusions listed below.

Conclusions

- Adequate methods exist for identifying chemical hazards in poultry and estimating their toxicity. Toxicological risks associated with a wide variety of chemicals, including herbicides, pesticides, food additives, and food and drinking water contaminants, have for several years been assessed on the basis of data obtained from experiments in animals. These methods of risk assessment can be used for chemical contaminants in poultry, although to date they have been applied primarily to other routes of exposure.

- The entry of chemical residues into poultry can be controlled with approaches adopted by the Environmental Protection Agency (EPA) and the Food and Drug Administration (FDA). These agencies have well-established procedures for systematically determining permissible levels of exposure to toxic chemicals and managing the points of entry of such substances into various types of environments. These procedures include such steps as establishing acceptable daily intakes, determining residue levels at which no observable toxic effects occur, and setting priorities based on the relative magnitude of various hazards. The toxicological data bases used by these agencies may not, however, be completely adequate to set limits for all chemical residues in poultry.

- A comprehensive approach to the control of chemical residues is not now possible. Of the four classes of chemicals categorized by the committee according to source, adequate data on occurrence exist for only one: chemicals that are intentionally added to poultry feed and water or are given to poultry to modify growth or prevent disease. Thus, there is a need to identify contaminants from several other sources and to determine which of them present the greatest potentially reducible risks and should therefore receive highest priority in a control program.
- Risks attributable to chemical residues in poultry should be assessed on a routine basis, because new chemicals may be introduced intentionally or accidentally into the environment at any time and because the data base is constantly growing. For example, there is a continual increase in information on the safety of environmental chemicals, especially on subchronic and chronic toxicity, on the basic biochemistry of toxicological effects, and on the relevance of toxic effects in animal models to humans.
- A comprehensive analysis of the risk of chemical residues in poultry was not possible, but in examining the limited data available the committee found no evidence that such residues pose a significant threat to public health.

Recommendations

The committee's major recommendations regarding chemical residues are based on its observation that important sources of residues are not considered in the FSIS monitoring program and that priorities for risk management are currently not set according to the relative magnitude of risk for known residues. If adopted by FSIS, the following recommendations should result in distinct improvements in the residue program:

- Using degree of risk as a basis, FSIS should establish priorities for monitoring residues and associated activities.
- Potentially hazardous chemical residues in poultry and their points of origin should be identified.
- The risks associated with identified hazardous residues should be determined.
- Using known risks as a basis, FSIS in collaboration with EPA and FDA should ensure that tolerance levels are set for known hazardous residues.
- Control programs to monitor the entry of residues into poultry should be developed.
- FSIS should determine how chemically contaminated poultry might

be removed from the marketplace or production line.

CURRENT FSIS PROGRAMS AND STATISTICALLY BASED SAMPLING

Current poultry inspection procedures focus primarily on the removal of diseased and damaged chickens, which are identified by organoleptic inspection techniques: observing, smelling, and feeling. These objectives, along with maintaining a sanitary environment, are valid components of any food-related quality assurance program, but should not be the only goals. This traditional approach to inspection can provide a foundation for the control of public health risks, but an effective program requires a broadened scope of activities based on quality assurance principles. Over several decades, detailed studies of quality assurance techniques in diverse fields of production and manufacture have shown that prevention of problems is the most effective means of controlling product quality. Such studies have shown that optimal product quality is most efficiently achieved through continuous monitoring based on a well-planned sampling protocol. A statistically based sampling scheme as part of a comprehensive quality assurance program for poultry would therefore offer advantages such as the following:

- Management of contamination by preventing its introduction at the source..
- Quick response to accidental contamination and the ability to trace defective birds to their sources.
- Continuous monitoring to observe the effects that result from adjusting variables in the program.
- Greater flexibility of data applications and more efficient use of resources.
- Application of data to quantitative risk assessments when necessary.
- Examination of birds, both macroscopically and microscopically, as dictated by need.

It should not be inferred that in such a program current inspection procedures would be applied to a smaller but more select sample of birds. Instead, a formal sampling system (as described in Chapter 7) necessarily involves more thorough examination of a well-defined but random group of birds; it might incorporate, for example, two conventional stages used continuously and a third stage for special programs, as follows:

In the first stage, a subset of birds could be randomly sampled and inspected in detail for general faults and gross disease. In the second stage, a smaller subsample could be randomly selected for more detailed study, including microbial load and simple chemical tests at the plant. In the third stage, a further random subsample of the second-stage sample could be frozen or otherwise preserved and sent to a central laboratory for studies not feasible at the plant, e.g., for testing in the National Residue Program. This final subsample should be subjected to morphologic and etiologic diagnoses to help build a data base against which future program activities can be measured. In each case, the rate of sampling and other details of the sampling process should be optimized on the basis of the best available information and the objectives of the inspection process. For example, the sampling rate might be periodically increased or decreased, depending on whether the results of previous samples and other information suggest an increase or decrease in the probability of encountering significant problems. The committee emphasizes, however, that less frequent but more intense examination of samples of chickens is not a substitute for maintaining a sanitary environment and that expert technical support and planning are required to ensure maximum benefits from such a program.

Conclusions

- The committee concluded that current procedures for selecting poultry samples for analysis of chemical contaminants are limited and are not sufficiently flexible to meet the needs of an expanding industry. For example, at the current monitoring rate of 300 samples per year, some plants may not be sampled for extended periods. Thus, even major problems might not be addressed in a timely manner.
- The current FSIS objective of ensuring a 95% probability of finding a chemical contaminant in a minimum of 1% of slaughtered poultry does not take into account the possibility of isolated accidental contaminations.
- Technical problems include lack of random sampling, absence of a system for continuous collection of data, lack of alternatives to simple random sampling (e.g., different rates of sampling, stratified random sampling), absence of flexibility to increase sample fractions under specific circumstances (e.g., when many birds are septicemic, when evisceration equipment malfunctions, or when a sampled bird dies of causes other than slaughter), and the inability to ensure that statistical variances are calculated correctly for data from complex samples.

Recommendations

- FSIS should begin to lay the groundwork for shifting resources from the organoleptic inspection of each broiler chicken to a more comprehensive program with statistically based sampling as one of its primary features. This should be undertaken as a first step in modifying the traditional bird-by-bird inspection system.
- FSIS should shift the focus of its residue program from the detection of contaminants in market-ready products to the prevention of their introduction at points as early as possible in the production process.
- Federal government support of broiler chicken inspection and related activities should be allocated primarily according to the degree that it can contribute to reductions in public health risk. The

current postmortem poultry inspection system does not address or meet this objective.
- A shift in the focus of FSIS programs toward the identification of contamination sources would necessarily extend the agency's interests to areas that are now the responsibility of other government (including state and local) agencies. FSIS should attempt to persuade such agencies that closer communication regarding poultry-associated health hazards is a matter of primary importance and that their effective control will require a concerted effort among responsible authorities.

The committee concluded, in agreement with the earlier Committee on the Scientific Basis of the Nation's Meat and Poultry Inspection Program, that FSIS should consider using risk-assessment techniques to manage and control poultry-associated hazards. Traditional poultry inspection techniques originated from the need to control diseases of poultry and to ensure a sanitary environment during slaughter. However, over the past few decades it has become apparent that the methods needed to detect and control poultry-associated public health threats are more complex than organoleptic inspection techniques alone can provide. The committee hopes that its risk model and its discussion of some potential applications will assist FSIS in controlling poultry-related health risks and developing a quality assurance program that will lead to nutritious and increasingly safe products.

Chapter 2

Poultry Inspection in the United States: History and Current Procedures

The current U.S. poultry inspection system can be traced to needs that first became apparent around the turn of the century. In the early 1900s, the poultry industry in the United States was little more than a sideline to farmers who raised fowl for personal consumption and sold some to bring their families a few extra dollars. Chickens and turkeys were mainly produced on small farms and sold, live or slaughtered, to local customers or transported to markets in the nearest cities. Farmers incubated, hatched, and brooded their own chicks using home-grown feeds and an assortment of remedies for disease. There were no standard poultry-raising methods, and the quality and quantity of poultry varied greatly from farm to farm. Furthermore, there were no government regulations to ensure the quality of poultry or other food products.

In 1906 the Meat Inspection Act was passed, but this legislation did not cover poultry. At that time and for a while afterward, poultry was a minor meat product, being regarded merely as a Sunday dinner speciality. Thus, small-scale production of poultry by independent farmers was adequate to meet public needs (USDA, 1984b). Most poultry was purchased by the consumer either live from the farmer-producer or a produce house or as a New York-dressed carcass (only blood and feathers removed). The housewife eviscerated and finally prepared the product for cooking, observing first-hand whether there were abnormalities, spoilage, or evidence of unwholesomeness (Libby, 1975).

As poultry production slowly increased, purchasers began to demand government inspection of live and slaughtered poultry. In the 1920s, there was an outbreak of avian influenza in New York City, which served as the major poultry distribution point. This incident led to an increased awareness of the need for ensuring product wholesomeness. As a result, cities, counties, and states began establishing their own inspection programs (USDA, 1984b).

In 1926, the Federal Poultry Inspection Service (FPIS) was established to assist localities in their inspection programs. In the beginning, FPIS inspected live poultry at railroad terminals and poultry markets in and around New York City. This voluntary inspection was conducted under an agreement between the U.S. Department of Agriculture (USDA) and two cooperating agencies—the New York Live Poultry Commission Merchants Association and the Greater New York Live Poultry Chamber of Commerce (USDA, 1984b). FPIS was also authorized to conduct its own voluntary postmortem inspection. Eviscerated poultry inspection was initiated by FPIS at the request of purchasers. Processors of canned goods containing poultry were frequently required by certain foreign and local governments to include FPIS wholesomeness certificates in all shipments of canned poultry products coming into their jurisdiction. Before 1940, most poultry was slaughtered and plucked in dressing plants and then shipped as New York-dressed poultry. Inspection was done at the point of delivery, if at all.

Military needs greatly increased the demand for poultry products during World War II, and military purchasing agents called on USDA to supply the inspection and certification services necessary for processors to meet military purchase specifications (USDA, 1984b). As military and consumer demand shifted from a preference for live poultry to New York-dressed poultry and then to ready-to-cook poultry, and as the industry attempted to accommodate these changes in demand, the USDA modified its inspection and certification program. Point-of-delivery inspection was not satisfactory for further processed products, such as ready-to-cook poultry, since the conditions of slaughtering and dressing would not be known by the consumer. For this reason, the military met its wartime poultry needs by purchasing only from plants that had been surveyed and found to meet military sanitation requirements. Soon thereafter, USDA required that evisceration and canning plants process New York-dressed poultry purchased only from plants that met USDA sanitation requirements.

USDA also established procedures for conducting antemortem inspections at the dressing plants. The formalization of these procedures accelerated a trend toward consolidating dressing and eviscerating activities within a single plant. During this period, inspection of poultry served two purposes: ensuring the wholesomeness of the poultry product and promoting sales by enabling processors to ship their product into jurisdictions that required certification. This dual role served to guide the federal government's voluntary poultry inspection program and provided the basis for passage of the Poultry Products Inspection Act (PPIA) in 1957 (USDA, 1984b).

PPIA required several kinds of inspection for poultry products destined for interstate commerce (USDA, 1984b):

- inspection of birds prior to slaughter
- inspection of each bird carcass after slaughter and before processing
- inspection of plant facilities to ensure sanitary conditions
- inspection of all slaughtering and processing operations
- verification of the truthfulness and accuracy of product labeling
- inspection of imported poultry products at the point of entry

This act also made mandatory the inspection of all poultry products intended for interstate commerce and thus subject to federal control. It required both antemortem inspection (to the extent deemed necessary by the USDA Secretary) and postmortem inspection of all birds slaughtered for such shipments, and sanitation inspection of all plants processing such products (USDA, 1984b).

The enactment of PPIA was not a response to perceived defects in the inspection system but, rather, a reaction to changes in consumer perceptions and marketing patterns. Poultry inspection activities during World War II increased consumer awareness of inspection. This in turn led to an increase in sales of poultry products bearing the FPIS certification mark. The fact that USDA certification was mahditory in order to market products in certain localities further stimulated industry interest in a broader federal inspection program. The substantial growth in the poultry industry during and immediately after the War had transformed it from one with primarily local markets to one with nationwide markets that could be effectively served only by uniform national inspection procedures and standards (USDA, 1984b).

The responsibility for implementing PPIA remained with the USDA's Agricultural Marketing Service (AMS), which had administered the voluntary poultry inspection program in effect before the Act was passed. AMS was strongly oriented toward facilitating the industry's ability to market agricultural commodities. Congress expressly recognized in its preamble to the PPIA the importance of marketing objectives as a basis for federal inspection, stating that:

> Unwholesome, adulterated, or misbranded poultry products impair the effective regulation of poultry products in interstate or foreign commerce, are injurious to the public welfare, destroy markets for wholesome, not adulterated, and properly labeled and packaged poultry products, and result in sundry losses to poultry producers and processors of poultry and poultry products, as well as injury to consumers (USC, 1983a, p. 833).

The Wholesome Poultry Products Act (WPPA) of 1968 required inspection of virtually all poultry sold to consumers. Previously, 16% of the chickens processed in the United States were not inspected by USDA because they were not transported across states lines and 31 states had no program of their own to cover the inspection of such poultry. The goal of the 1968 Act was to bring this uninspected poultry under an inspection program, whether state or federally operated (USDA, 1984b). The Act established federal-state cooperative programs of inspection closely paralleling those established under the Wholesome Meat Act passed a year earlier. The federal government supplied technical assistance and up to 50% of the funding for state-approved inspection programs. To gain such support, state programs had to establish requirements at least equal to those of the federal inspection program. The 1968 Act also required USDA to take ovar the inspection programs of states that did not develop an acceptable program within a specified period (USDA, 1984b).

Although WPPA ammended the 1957 PPIA, no significant changes were made in federal antemortem or postmortem inspection processes. Antemortem inspections continued on samples obtained from flocks, whereas postmortem inspection of each bird remained mandatory. No major changes have been made in the poultry inspection laws since 1968 (USDA, 1984b), despite the more than tripling of the pounds of poultry inspected (see Table 2-1).

TABLE 2-1. History of Inspected Plants[a]

Year	Number of Plants	Live Weight of Birds Inspected (billions of pounds)
1927	1	Not available
1928	7	0.0032
1940	35	0.076
1954	260	1.0
1958	468	2.0
1964	201	6.6
1975	154	13.7
1981	371	20.0

[a] From USDA, 1984b.

POULTRY INSPECTION ACTIVITIES

To meet its statutory requirements under PPIA, the USDA administers at least eight public health-related inspection activities:

antemortem inspection
postmortem inspection
condemnation and final disposition
sanitary slaughter and dressing
poultry chilling
plant sanitation
carcass reinspection
residue monitoring

Brief descriptions of each public health-related activity specified by PPIA are provided in the following paragraphs:

Antemortem Inspection

According to the PPIA,

The Secretary shall, where and to the extent considered by him necessary, cause to be made by inspectors antemortem inspection of poultry in each official establishment processing poultry or poultry products for commerce . . . . (USC, 1983b, p. 838).

Antemortem inspection (USDA, 1984b) refers to the examination of live poultry to detect signs of disease. The USDA inspector observes the flocks between the time they arrive at the slaughtering plant and the time birds are hung on the slaughtering line. Because antemortem inspection is discretionary, it is conducted not bird by bird but on samples selected from flocks or groups of birds in their crates. At times, however, the inspector may examine individual birds to investigate clinical signs and to judge body temperature, fleshing, and state of hydration.

Antemortem inspection may result in a bird being passed for subsequent delivery to the consumer, condemned, or designated as suspect. A bird is condemned if it plainly shows evidence of any disease or condition that would cause condemnation of its carcass during postmortem inspection. Birds that have already died are automatically condemned. Condemned birds may not be processed further, nor may they be conveyed into any area of the plant where other poultry or poultry products are held or prepared. They must be disposed of in a prescribed manner (USDA, 1984b).

A bird is designated as suspect if it appears to be affected with any condition that may cause condemnation during postmortem inspection. Birds so classified are segregated from other poultry and held for separate slaughter, evisceration, and postmortem inspection (USDA, 1984b).

Most producers augment the USDA process with their own antemortem inspection programs, primarily to provide the plant with early data on probable flock condemnation rates. At present, antemortem inspection accounts for less than 1% of a USDA inspector's inspection activities (USDA, 1984b).

Postmortem Inspection

Bird-by-bird postmortem inspection of carcasses is required for all poultry slaughtered in a federally inspected establishment. Inspectors observe the carcass exterior; open the body cavity and examine inner surfaces and organs, including the liver, heart, spleen, and other viscera; and instruct a trimmer (a plant employee) on the disposition of each carcass. This inspection is designed to ensure that each bird is free from readily apparent disease (such as leukosis, septicemia, toxemia, air sacculitis, tumors, and parasites), that it is not badly bruised or otherwise damaged, and that it did not die from any cause other than slaughter (USDA, 1984b).

Following is a list of the manual operations required for the traditional method of postmortem inspection as described by Libby and Humphreys (1975):

Right-hand operation:

Grasp one leg, run hand down leg to determine indication of bone disease.
Open body cavity to view internal surfaces.
Turn body to view outside of bird (including head) for disease, abnormalities, and dressing imperfections.

Left-hand operation:

Place hand over liver to feel for consistency, texture, and lesions, viewing simultaneously.
Slip fingers around liver and grasp the spleen between thumb and finger, rolling spleen to determine texture and presence of abnormal condition. In case of fryers and broilers it is not necessary to roll spleen. Simultaneously view other viscera while checking spleen. A differing opening cut (i.e., along back) may require slight modifications in this procedure (Libby and Humphreys, 1975, pp. 170-171).

To facilitate inspection and prevent contamination of edible tissues, PPIA requires that the carcass be presented in such a way that the entire carcass, including the internal and external body surfaces and all the internal organs, can be thoroughly inspected (Libby and Humphreys, 1975). Hocks must be cut in preparation for inspection so that the telltale exudates of infectious synovitis in tendon sheaths and joint capsules can be detected. The feet are removed just before the inspection and, in all cases, after the carcasses have passed the last washer unit. Washing the carcass after cutting of the hocks would of course interfere with this inspection. The heads of young chickens can be removed prior to inspection. The heads of mature chickens may be removed before postmortem inspection, provided the inspector in charge has determined at antemortem inspection that such removal will not affect postmortem disposition. Permission to remove the heads from a particular group or lot of mature chickens may be rescinded by the inspector in charge, or a designee, if the the heads are needed to make a proper disposition.

Plants are also required to provide certain facilities at the inspection station. For example, a switch or button control must be accessible to the inspector, who can then stop or start the processing line in connection with postmortem and sanitation control. In addition, adequate lighting of uniform intensity must be provided at all working levels. Plants are also required to separate double lines of carcasses with dividers to prevent confusion and to ensure that each carcass will receive the inspector's attention. Visceral organs must be placed near the carcass from which they have been removed. Hand-washing facilities must be adequate and properly located at both operating and inspecting positions (Libby and Humphreys, 1975).

A trained company employee called a trimmer must be assigned to each inspector to perform such functions as plucking feathers, trimming bruises, moving condemned birds from the shackles into condemned cans, placing suspect birds on the hang-back rack for more detailed inspection by the Veterinary Medical Officer (VMO), marking the condemnation record sheet, and generally assisting the inspector in routines related to the inspection procedures. Production lines must be adequately staffed with properly trained employees functioning under effective supervision (Libby and Humphreys, 1975).

Condemnation and Final Disposition

On the basis of the inspector's postmortem examination, birds are passed, trimmed and passed, retained for disposition by the VMO, or condemned for any of 11 different reasons (see Table 2-2). The inspector has only 2 to 3 seconds to examine each bird and to decide its disposition (USDA, 1984b). In this manner more than 4.7 billion birds were inspected in fiscal year 1984 (USDA, 1985).

Sanitary Slaughter and Dressing

The principal objective of sanitary dressing is to defeather the bird and to remove its gastrointestinal tract and other internal organs with minimal contamination of edible tissues. In many cases localized or generalized diseases, infections, or contaminations are not detected until the dressing operation has been partially or entirely completed.

Preventing fecal contamination of the carcass from spillage of gastrointestinal contents or smearing of external fecal matter on outer skin surfaces is the single most important aspect of sanitary slaughter and dressing. Ideally, slaughter and dressing should be designed to reduce or preferably eliminate contamination from this source.

Poultry Chilling

After inspection, ready-to-cook poultry is promptly chilled or frozen at temperatures that inhibit microbial growth. All slaughtered and eviscerated birds are chilled to an internal temperature of 40°F (4°C) or less within 4 hours (for a 4-lb. bird), 6 hours (for a 4to 8-lb. bird), or 8 hours (for a carcass heavier than 8 lbs.) unless they are to be frozen or cooked immediately at the establishment. FSIS has responsibility for ensuring that these chilling specifications are met.

TABLE 2-2. Number and Percentage of Young Chickens (Broilers) Condemned during Postmortem Inspection, by Cause, in Fiscal Year 1984[a]

Cause of Condemnation>	Number Condemned	Percent of Total Inspected[b]
Tuberculosis	0	0
Leukosis	2,056,872	0.05
Septicemia	15,111,696	0.36
Air sacculitis	8,087,665	0.19
Synovitis	267,528	0.01
Tumors	1,394,009	0.03
Bruises	735,353	0.02
Cadaver	1,544,661	0.04
Contamination	2,371,952	0.06
Overscald	528,282	0.01
Other	1,496.702	0.04
TOTAL	33,594,720	0.81

[a] From USDA, 1985.

[b] in FY1984, 4,203,133,000 broilers were inspected. This represents 89% of all poultry slaughtered (4,722,839,000) in the United States during that period.

Packed poultry held at the plant for more than 24 hours must be kept at 36°F (2°c) or less. Giblets are chilled to 40°F (4°c) or lower within 2 hours from the time they are removed from the inedible viscera, except when they are cooled with the carcass (CFR, 1983). Only potable water may be used for ice and water chilling. The ice is handled and stored in a sanitary manner; block ice is washed by spraying all surfaces with clean water before crushing (NRC, 1985).

Plant Sanitation

Inspection of the sanitation practices of poultry plants begins in the poultry holding areas and continues through the handling of live birds, their carcasses, and the products derived from them. The inspectors examine structural aspects of the premises, water supply, manure and sewage disposal, equipment, personnel, and other features of the plant environment (Blair, 1975).

Slaughtering or processing in an unclean environment or under unclean conditions is prohibited—a requirement that is enforced by the inspector's ability to reject an unclean department or piece of equipment. The plant is warned that the department or equipment identified must not be placed in service until it has been made acceptable and released for use by the inspector (Blair, 1975). In addition, the inspector completes a daily sanitation report (MP Form 455, August 1979) that covers such items as plant cleanliness, rodent and insect control, ice facilities, and dry storage areas. A copy of the daily report is provided to the establishment.

Carcass Reinspection

After dressing operations and routine postmortem inspection are completed, selected samples of chickens are reinspected according to a preestablished sampling plan. Defects are evaluated on the basis of accept-reject criteria, and the result is extended to all carcasses represented by the sample. The Acceptable Quality Level (AQL) standards developed in 1973 (USDA, 1974) are applied in all poultry plants with traditional and modified traditional inspection procedures (Berndt, 1985) to detect dressing defects in broiler carcasses after chilling. The data collected include information on the origin, extent, and nature of carcass contamination so that corrective action can be initiated at the source (USDA, 1983a).

Recently, FSIS introduced Finished Product Standards (FPS), which make use of the Cumulative Sum System (CUSUM) to score the presence of defects such as ingesta, feces, feathers, grease, bile remnants, blisters, bruises, sores, scabs, and other lesions on birds. In this system, defects in a sample of carcasses are counted both before and after chilling. Birds not meeting the standards are "determined by the FSIS to be adulterated" (Anonymous, 1986b, p. 4). The FPS were developed from data obtained from a random sampling survey of trim and processing defects in 25 poultry plants. In 1983 and 1984 the results of this survey were compared to AQL in eight pilot poultry plants, and the two sets of standards proved to be comparable (Berndt, 1985).

Residue Monitoring

In 1967, the National Residue Program (NRP) was established in FSIS. This program is the U.S. Government's principal regulatory mechanism for determining the presence and level of chemicals in poultry judged, primarily by the Food and Drug Administration (FDA), the Environmental Protection Agency (EPA), and FSIS, to be of public health concern. (FDA and EPA prescribe the conditions under which approved drugs are allowed in poultry). Through this program, FSIS applies new technologies and testing procedures in the monitoring of approximately 100 of the chemicals that may be found in poultry and red meat. FSIS uses an advisory board of scientists from FDA, EPA, and

FSIS to select these chemicals on the basis of their toxicity, exposure levels, persistence, and other relevant criteria (USDA, 1986).

The NRP has four major objectives: monitoring, surveillance, exploratory testing, and prevention of chemical residues in poultry (USDA, 1984a). These objectives are described in the following paragraphs.

Monitoring. Monitoring is accomplished through random sampling of imported poultry products and tissues from apparently healthy poultry as they pass through routine inspection at slaughter (postmortem inspection). These samples are tested for compliance with chemical tolerance levels and are studied to determine patterns and trends in the distribution, frequency, and levels of chemical residues and to identify tolerance-or action-level violations. For example, approximately 7,500 domestic samples and 434 samples of imported poultry products were scheduled for such testing in 1986 (USDA, 1986).

Poultry tested under the monitoring system is normally sold and consumed before test results are available. The findings are referred to FDA or EPA for review and for use in on-the-farm inspections to determine whether chemicals are misused. On occasion, test results can trigger surveillance testing.

Chemicals are periodically added to or deleted from a test list of approximately 100 chemicals. Some monitoring is designed to discern the presence of so-called generic components. For example, the presence of any member of the family of arsenicals is determined by testing for the presence of arsenic. In general, the number of samples selected for the testing of one chemical is designed to ensure, at the 95% confidence level, that the chemical will be detected in at least one sample if it occurs with a uniform distribution in 1% or more of the population of birds slaughtered during a given year.

Surveillance. Surveillance is achieved by targeted sampling of poultry products to control or investigate suspected violations. Approximately 7,200 domestic samples, including poultry, and no samples of imported products were scheduled for surveillance in 1986 (USDA, 1986). Surveillance testing may be initiated when a producer is suspected of marketing animals with residues above limits set by EPA or FDA. Carcasses are retained while the tests are conducted. If violations are found, the carcasses are condemned and the producer is instructed not to market other birds until additional tissue samples no longer contain illegal residues.

Before poultry products can be imported into the United States, the countries of origin must monitor them for residues in programs similar to those in effect in this country. When these products reach their U.S. port of entry, they are once again randomly tested for residues.

Exploratory Testing. In exploratory testing, random or nonrandom samples of poultry are taken to study chemicals for which safe limits have not been established (e.g., mycotoxins, trace chemicals, or industrial chemicals). The information gained from these tests is used to define the distribution of the chemicals as well as the frequency and levels of their occurrence. The exploratory program also includes studies to help develop new methods for evaluating existing programs.

Prevention of Chemical Residues. In collaboration with USDA's Extension Service, FSIS initiated a chemical residue prevention program in 1981. This program is designed to help domestic poultry producers prevent chemical contamination of their birds. It is a primarily educational undertaking that provides counseling by extension service personnel and consulting specialists (USDA, 1983b).

CHANGING ENVIRONMENT FOR POULTRY PRODUCTION AND REGULATION

In the years since the establishment of the basic principles of poultry inspection, a growing population and changing consumer tastes have caused rapid growth in the poultry industry. Increasing demand along with technological advances have produced a consolidated, vertically integrated, and highly competitive industry. To meet the new demands for a wide range of products at an acceptable cost, processors have adopted new techniques and innovative processing methods. Poultry are now bred and raised in environments to promote growth and prevent disease. The controlled use of vaccines and drugs, such as antibiotics, has greatly improved the health of the birds and decreased the number rejected at inspection as unfit for human consumption. Quality control systems have increased the poultry producers' ability to deliver uniform, high-quality flocks to the slaughterhouse. Poultry slaughtering and processing have largely been automated, and faster, more systematic procedures have replaced less-standardized, manual operations. Advances in packaging and preservation have reduced the likelihood of chemical or microbiological contamination.

Poultry production and processing has become a highly concentrated industry. Today, about 20 companies operate approximately 220 broiler chicken plants (USDA, 1983c), and 5% of these plants account for almost 65% of the total production. Poultry slaughtering has also become more concentrated—42% of the plants slaughter 75% of all broilers. Vertical integration has enhanced industry control over the raising and slaughtering of birds. Approximately 95% of all poultry producers control their birds' entire life cycles. The increased use of brand names, which are now given to 65% of all poultry products sold at retail, along with the growing selectivity of consumers and potential legal liability have provided strong motivation for quality control on the part of producers.

The inherent quality of poultry products has undoubtedly improved, but progress in reducing the public health hazards associated with poultry has not been entirely uniform. The proliferation of environmental contaminants and chemicals added to poultry feeds and, to some extent, processed foods has increased the possibility that potentially harmful chemical residues will be found in poultry.

The production of poultry products has also become more complex. Early in this century, only a few basic cuts of poultry were available. At present, there is great variety of raw, canned, cured, dried, fermented, and frozen products. Any aesthetic benefits derived from this variety are sometimes offset by new sources of food-borne microbial organisms and chemicals and opportunities for them to contaminate the products. Thus, public health concerns now include antibiotic-resistant bacteria as well as chemical toxicity. Currently, eight broad classes of public health risk are of concern in poultry inspection: bacteria, bacterial toxins, parasites, fungal toxins, viruses, toxic chemical residues, intentional additives, and process-associated toxicants (NRC, 1985).

Increased poultry production coupled with inflation has led to a substantial rise in the cost of inspection. Because of these factors, the labor-intensive nature of postmortem inspection, and the regulatory requirement to inspect each bird, taxpayer costs for the present kind of inspection may be expected to continue to increase proportionately with the industry growth rate.

By law, the federal government provides all inspection services and pays for all inspection except overtime and holiday work requested by slaughtering establishments. As inspection costs have escalated, FSIS program managers have been under increased pressure to justify their programs and to make them more efficient. Furthermore, all regulatory agencies have been asked to eliminate unnecessary regulatory burdens to facilitate improvements in productivity (Presidential Documents, 1981).

These changes in disease prevalence, poultry husbandry, and financial resources have encouraged FSIS to develop more efficient inspection techniques and procedures that will increase, or at least not lower, health protection. For example, one change instituted in the mid-1970s is the development and testing of alternative postmortem inspection procedures that partially shift the burden for maintaining the quality of inspected poultry from FSIS to plant management working under FSIS supervision.

ALTERNATIVE POSTMORTEM POULTRY INSPECTION PROCEDURES

Postmortem inspection procedures, the most labor-intensive aspect of inspection, have been the principal targets of efforts to increase efficiency. These procedures have recently been modified by FSIS to increase production efficiency and decrease production time, and further changes are being explored (FSIS, 1984; FSIS, personal communication, 1984).

As noted above, traditional postmortem inspection procedures require a complete examination of each slaughtered bird and all its parts, including a relatively cumbersome sequence of hand motions to manipulate each carcass (Berndt, 1985). In 1979 FSIS instituted a less labor-intensive method called the Modified Traditional Inspection (MTI) system (FSIS, personal communication, 1984). Under MTI, three inspectors work in sequence to inspect each bird. One inspector examines the outside surfaces of each carcass, using a mirror to see the back of the bird. The other two inspectors examine the inside surfaces and viscera, coordinating their actions so that each handles every other bird. The hand motions for inspecting the inside of the carcass and its internal organs were also redesigned and streamlined. The MTI system was tested in the field and found to be more efficient than and as effective as the traditional system in identifying evaluated abnormalities. Maximum line speed achievable under MTI is 70 birds per minute (FSIS, 1984).

FSIS has explored and begun to adopt several other methods of sequenced inspection. One method, known as the hands on/hands off procedure (FSIS, personal communication, 1984), involves a team of four inspectors. The first one examines the outside surfaces of a carcass; the second examines the drawn viscera, which are hung on another line. Both inspectors use mirrors, not their hands. The birds are then alternately assigned to the other two inspectors, who examine the inside surfaces with their hands. This procedure is now used in only two broiler plants in the United States (Berndt, 1985).

In a similar, even less labor-intensive design called the total hands-off procedure, a machine opens the carcasses for inside viewing. The inspector does not touch either the internal organs or the carcass. Because initial tests indicate that this system is not as effective as the traditional and MTI inspection procedures, it has not been implemented. Future use of this approach will require either the development of improved equipment for opening the birds effectively and consistently so that the inspectors have an unobstructed view, or a change in the criteria used to judge the effectiveness of inspection.

In 1982, FSIS began field trials of the New Line Speed (NELS) inspection system, a quality control system operated by the plant but monitored by an FSIS inspector (Berndt, 1985; FSIS, 1984). Under NELS, the government inspectors inspect the birds and determine which birds should be condemned and which should be passed for food. The plant workers then inspect the passed birds for certain outside defects, which they trim. Eliminating the need for direct FSIS participation in the trimming of each carcass reduces inspector time per carcass. With NELS, the maximum line speed depends on a plant's ability to provide inspectors with properly presented birds. As the proportion of defective birds increases, line speeds necessarily decrease. Presently, 10 U.S. plants are using NELS on a test basis. Most of these plants operate line speeds of approximately 90 birds per minute.

In 1985 FSIS made further departures from traditional inspection by testing a system that would transfer responsibilities for all bird inspection to plant personnel working under a plant-operated quality control system (Berndt, 1985). In this Third-Generation Inspection System, the government's role is limited to inspection of a sample of birds to ensure that the quality control system is working properly. Two FSIS inspectors are stationed on each production line. One of them sets a standard for inspection by which five industry inspectors, who have been trained and certified in the NELS procedure, are judged. An automated computer system compares each plant inspector's level of performance (in terms of frequency of inspection actions) to that of the USDA food inspector and indicates, through light and audio alarms, when performance is questionable. The second government inspector, who is stationed at the end of the line, uses that information to compare the condemnation and trim rates of the industry inspectors with those of the USDA standard-setter and initiates specific action to respond to any problem. This last inspector also looks for abnormalities suggesting the need for condemnation of birds at the end of the line where the birds pass at a rate of 182 birds per minute. FSIS claims that this final step meets the legal requirements for bird-by-bird inspection (Berndt, 1985).

Recently, FSIS embarked on a program to modify MTI, still the most widely used postmortem inspection system, by incorporating some features found to be effective in the other systems it has explored. In the new system, called the Streamlined Inspection System (SIS) (Anonymous, 1986b), one or two inspectors (SIS-1 or SIS-2) are needed instead of the three used in MTI, depending on the size of the plant. Each inspector will examine the whole bird, i.e., the outside of birds and the inside cavities and internal organs. A plant employee termed a helper and assigned to each inspector will identify bruises, broken wings, and other manufacturing defects to be trimmed by other plant employees after the giblets are removed. This assistance will allow FSIS inspectors to concentrate on detecting diseases and other abnormalities. In addition to obtaining new equipment and making some facility changes (Anonymous, 1986b; FSIS, 1986), the 137 plants now using MTI will be required to maintain an FPS program that includes a prechill test to measure the effectiveness of processing controls and a postchill test to measure changes (such as moisture absorption) that take place during the chilling process. The CUSUM statistical sampling method (see above section on Carcass Reinspection) will be used by FSIS to monitor the adequacy of plant trimming and processing operations to ensure that the product meets regulatory standards (Anonymous, 1986a). The maximum line speeds on SIS will be 35 birds per minute under one inspector and 70 birds per minute under two inspectors, the same rate now allowed for the three inspectors under MTI.

CONCERNS REGARDING THE HEALTH IMPACTS OF NEW INSPECTION SYSTEMS

According to public opinion polls, the general population apparently has confidence that the current traditional system of poultry inspection is sufficiently adequate to ensure that poultry products reaching the marketplace are as safe and wholesome as is technically feasible (Good Housekeeping Institute, 1983; Roper Organization, Inc., 1983). However, some of the recently adopted and proposed changes in the poultry inspection programs have been perceived by the public, consumer advocates, and inspection staff as compromising human health and safety (Community Nutrition Institute, 1977; Hughes, 1983). The changes that produce or could produce substantial increases in line speed have drawn the most criticism. Also of concern are the health effects of low-level contamination of poultry by pesticides, drugs, and environmental contaminants—none of which can be found by organoleptic inspection. Meanwhile, the industry has questioned the necessity and efficiency of 100% postmortem inspection (i.e., the inspection of every bird) in groups of poultry that are almost uniformly in good health (NRC, 1984).

FSIS contends that none of the changes made to date have reduced the effectiveness of the poultry inspection program. Further major efficiencies will almost certainly require a move toward the inspection of only a sample of birds. Intense inspection of a sample combined with an industry shift from detection of problems to their prevention would have many advantages. However, FSIS may have difficulty persuading the general public (as well as its own inspection staff) that a sampling system based on a substantially more intense inspection of some sample of products could in fact lead to better identification of problem areas and hence improve public health protection.

The Need for Risk Assessment

In 1984, recognizing the need to evaluate new and proposed changes to meat and poultry inspection procedures in general, FSIS asked the Food and Nutrition Board (FNB) to examine the scientific basis of USDA's meat and poultry inspection program. The committee appointed to perform that task concluded that the new postmortem inspection procedures for poultry instituted between 1979 and 1983 "are not likely to diminish protection of the public health," but noted that it could make no overall assessment of risks and benefits because it could find no comprehensive statement of criteria, no systematic accumulation of data, and no complete technical analysis of the hazards or benefits to human health in the traditional inspection program or as a consequence of the adoption of new techniques (NRC, 1985, pp. 7-8).

That committee considered whether to recommend the newly proposed cooperative industry-government inspection system for chickens, in which the USDA inspector's primary responsibility is to monitor inspection performed by plant personnel. It concluded, "No such change should be recommended until a detailed risk analysis, based on sound scientific data, compares the present and proposed approaches and documents that efforts of FSIS to attain its major public health objective would not be harmed" (NRC, 1985, p. 91). The committee also recommended that FSIS establish a risk-assessment program to help organize and evaluate its risk-management strategies. Through such a program, FSIS could establish limits on the concentrations of chemical residues that can be tolerated in poultry products, set priorities for controlling residues, and design programs to ensure compliance with established limits.

The report prepared by the committee pointed to two key elements that are missing from the present FSIS approach to inspection and risk management: comprehensive assessment of the kinds of public health hazards that face the U.S. public and objective criteria to determine whether solutions to identified problems are being appropriately and successfully pursued. The committee recommended that FSIS apply formal risk-assessment procedures to assist in the planning and evaluation of all phases of poultry inspection, especially in the assessment of public health consequences that might result from modification of the inspection process.

In response to the committee's observations, the FSIS Administrator asked the FNB to undertake another study with two goals: analysis of the public health risks associated with broiler chickens at the time of slaughter and development of methods for comparing the effects on public health of different inspection goals and strategies. The findings of that study are described in this report.

REFERENCES

Anonymous. 1986a. Equipment for SIS. Natl. Provis. 194:5.

Anonymous. 1986b. Streamlined Inspection System (SIS). Fed. Vet. 43:3-4.

Berndt, D. L. 1985. Response to NAS Committee Questions. Slaughter Inspection Standards and Procedures Division, Meat and Poultry Inspection Technical Services, Food Safety and Inspection Service, U.S. Department of Agriculture, Washington, D.C. 14 pp.

Blair, J. L. 1975. Elements and controls of meat hygiene. Pp. 16-32 in J. A. Libby, ed. Meat Hygiene, 4th ed. Lea & Febiger, Philadelphia.

CFR (Code of Federal Regulations). 1983. Title 9, Animals and Animal Products; Section 381.66, Temperatures and chilling and freezing procedures. U.S. Government Printing Office, Washington, D.C.

Community Nutrition Institute. 1977. Assessment of the Booz-Allen & Hamilton, Inc., Study and Recommendations on a Reorganization of the Meat and Poultry Inspection Program. Community Nutrition Institute, Washington, D.C. [35 pp.]

FSIS (Food Safety and Inspection Service). 1984. New line speed inspection system for broilers and cornish hens. Proposed rule. Docket No. 82-023P. Fed. Regist. 49:2473-2478.

FSIS (Food Safety and Inspection Service). 1986. Facility and equipment requirements for the Streamlined Inspection System for broilers and cornish game hens. Proposed rule. Docket No. 85-036P. Fed. Regist. 51:3621-3624.

Good Housekeeping Institute. 1983. Food Labeling Study. Consumer Research Department, Good Housekeeping Institute, New York. 38 pp.

Hughes, K. 1983. Return to the Jungle: How the Reagan Administration is Imperiling the Nation's Meat and Poultry Inspection Program. Center for the Study of Responsive Law, Washington, D.C. 63 pp.

Libby, J. A. 1975. History. Pp. 1-15 in J. A. Libby, ed. Meat Hygiene, 4th ed. Lea & Febiger, Philadelphia.

Libby, J. A., and M. R. Humphreys. 1975. Post-mortem dispositions. Pp. 85-186 in J. A. Libby, ed. Meat Hygiene, 4th ed. Lea & Febiger, Philadelphia.

NRC (National Research Council). 1984. Transcript of Public Meeting. Committee on the Scientific Basis for Meat and Poultry Inspection Programs. On file with the Food and Nutrition Board, Washington, D.C. 81 pp.

NRC (National Research Council). 1985. Meat and Poultry Inspection: The Scientific Basis of the Nation's Program. Report of the Committee on the Scientific Basis of the Nation's Meat and Poultry Inspection Program, Food and Nutrition Board. National Academy Press, Washington, D.C. 209 pp.

Presidential Documents. 1981. Executive Order 12291 of February 17, 1981—Federal Regulation. Fed. Regist. 46:13193-13198.

Roper Organization, Inc. 1983. Postal service most favored of federal departments. P. 2 in Roper Reports, Summary of 83-5. Roper Organization, New York.

USC (U.S. Code). 1983a. Title 21, Food and Drugs; Section 451, Congressional statement of findings. United States Code, 1982 ed. U.S. Government Printing Office, Washington, D.C.

USC (U.S. Code). 1983b. Title 21, Food and Drugs; Section 455, Inspection in official establishments. United States Code, 1982 ed. U.S. Government Printing Office, Washington, D.C.

USDA (U.S. Department of Agriculture). 1974. MPI Directive 918.1, Poultry Carcass Inspection Program. MPI Bulletin 619, issued February 25, 1974. Meat and Poultry Inspection Program, Animal and Plant Health Inspection Service, U.S. Department of Agriculture, Washington, D.C. 2 pp.

USDA (U.S. Department of Agriculture). 1983a. Meat and Poultry Inspection Manual, Combined Changes 83-1 through 83-12. Meat and Poultry Inspection, Food Safety and Inspection Service, U.S. Department of Agriculture, Washington, D.C. [37 pp.]

USDA (U.S. Department of Agriculture). 1983b. Prevention—A new direction in reducing the risk of chemical residues in meat and poultry. Pp. 21-23 in Food Safety and Inspection Service Program Plan: Fiscal Year 1984. Food Safety and Inspection Service, U.S. Department of Agriculture, Washington, D.C.

USDA (U.S. Department of Agriculture). 1983c. Protection and Productivity: The Strategy for Meat and Poultry Inspection in the 1980's. Food Safety and Inspection Service, U.S. Department of Agriculture, Washington, D.C. 40 pp.

USDA (U.S. Department of Agriculture). 1984a. FSIS Facts: The National Residue Program. FSIS-18. Food Safety and Inspection Service, U.S. Department of Agriculture, Washington, D.C. 4 pp.

USDA (U.S. Department of Agriculture). 1984b. A Review of the Slaughter Regulations under the Poultry Products Inspection Act. Regulations Office, Policy and Program Planning, Food Safety and Inspection Service, U.S. Department of Agriculture, Washington, D.C. 28 pp.

USDA (U.S. Department of Agriculture). 1985. Statistical Summary: Federal Meat and Poultry Inspection for Fiscal Year 1984. FSIS-14. Food Safety and Inspection Service, U.S. Department of Agriculture, Washington, D.C. 39 pp.

USDA (U.S. Department of Agriculture). 1986. Compound Evaluation and Analytical Capability: Annual Residue Plan. Science Program, Food Safety and Inspection Service, U.S. Department of Agriculture, Washington, D.C. 127 pp.

Chapter 3

Risk-Assessment Model for Poultry Inspection: Analytical Approach

As indicated in Chapter 2, it is generally accepted that the design and selection of inspection strategies for controlling human health risks associated with broiler chickens should be based on risk assessment. The present committee concluded that a complete quantitative risk assessment is not possible at this time because of a lack of data and limited resources. However, a qualitative assessment based on the concepts of risk assessment and the judgments of experts can be done. An analytical approach developed by the committee to conduct such an assessment is described in this chapter.

OVERVIEW OF THE ANALYTICAL APPROACH

The analytical approach recommended for the conduct and application of risk assessment requires first a conceptual framework and second, a risk model. For its conceptual framework, the committee adopted the well-accepted view of the role and nature of risk assessment developed in 1983 by the National Research Council's Committee on the Institutional Means for Assessment of Risks to Public Health. That committee proposed that risk assessment proceed in four steps (NRC, 1983):

- Hazard identification: Determination, based on qualitative and quantitative evidence, of whether a particular agent (e.g., a chemical or microorganism) is or is not causally linked to particular health effects.
- Dose-response assessment: Determination of the relationship between the magnitude of exposure and the probability that a given health effect will occur.
- Exposure assessment: Determination of the extent of human exposure before or after application of regulatory controls.
- Risk characterization: Description of the nature and often the magnitude of human risk, including attendant uncertainty.

Important in this conceptual framework is the relationship between risk management and these four steps of risk assessment. The 1983 risk assessment committee reported that:

Regulatory actions are based on two distinct elements, <u>risk assessment</u> . . . and <u>risk management</u>. Risk assessment is the use of the factual base to define the health effects of exposure of individuals or populations to hazardous materials and situations. Risk management is the process of weighing policy alternatives and selecting the most appropriate regulatory action, integrating the results of risk assessment with engineering data and with social, economic, and political concerns to reach a decision (NRC, 1983, p. 3).

This concept leads to two important conclusions. First, the primary purpose of risk assessment is to support decisions regarding regulatory actions. Although there are nonregulatory uses of risk assessment corresponding to the full range of nonregulatory options for risk management, the regulatory orientation of the above quotation is appropriate to the responsibility of FSIS. The second conclusion is derived from the first and from the desire that risk assessments not prejudice or mislead decision makers. That is, to the greatest extent possible, risk assessments should be devoid of value judgments. Judgments are needed in risk assessment, but they should be judgments of science unbiased by the scientist's preferences for specific risk-management policies.

Partitioning risk assessment into four standardized steps helps to ensure that there is a comprehensive accounting of the factors that determine risk and minimizes the policy and value judgments that might otherwise be inserted into the analysis. The key to risk characterization, the final step in the risk-assessment process, is the development and application of a risk model that guides the analyst in integrating and drawing conclusions from the first three steps: identification of the hazard, dose-response assessments, and exposure assessment.

In a formal, quantitative risk assessment, the risk model consists of equations and mathematical algorithms and is often implemented as a computer code. These equations and algorithms may be developed to varying degrees of rigor, depending on the problem and the needs of the user. For qualitative risk assessment, the risk model is not formalized to permit rigorous numerical calculations. A qualitative model does, however, identify possible sources of risk and how they might be linked to health effects, and thus can be a valuable tool. By using such a model, investigators can conduct a formal review of the data demonstrating that a hazard exists, and organize information on dose-response relationships and exposures. Qualitative models are useful because they provide a logical framework for asking specific questions and deriving conclusions systematically. Qualitative risk assessment is essential before quantitative risk assessment can be undertaken.

A model to determine the risks of a process as complicated as poultry production and consumption must disaggregate the complex processes leading to the generation of those risks. The model must take into consideration points in the process at which hazard or risk agents are introduced into poultry or poultry products and modification of the quantities or characteristics of these agents by subsequent steps in the process. It can then be used to identify and determine the logical interrelationships of important critical factors that control the level of risk—that is, activities and events that introduce, alter, or determine the size of human health risks.

In developing a model to assess the human health risks associated with poultry, the committee reviewed the principal risk agents associated with poultry production and consumption. These are summarized below and are described in more detail in Chapters 4 and 5.

POULTRY RISK AGENTS

The agents responsible for nearly all the human health risks arising during the production and consumption of broiler chickens fall into two categories:

- Pathogenic microorganisms or their toxins. These agents, such as various species of <u>Salmonella</u> and <u>Campylobacter</u>, can transmit diseases to humans when present in or on infected or contaminated poultry tissues.
- Poultry-borne chemical residues. As described in Chapter 2, residues maybe found in poultry intentionally given or exposed in other ways to chemicals before slaughter. After exposure, these chemicals may be concentrated and retained in the tissues for long periods.

THE RISK MODEL

In general, risk is dependent on the existence of three factors:

- A source from which risk agents are generated or released into the environment. For poultry production and consumption, the risk source encompasses all the activities related to poultry production, slaughtering, and processing.
- A route of human exposure to the risk agents, e.g., distribution and consumption of poultry products.
- A mechanism by which the exposures can generate adverse health effects, e.g., through microbial and chemical factors, which determine the health consequences resulting from human consumption or other contact with poultry products.

A risk model may be developed by identifying and linking all significant influences on these three factors.

Figure 3-1 shows the major components, or submodels, of the risk model. Figures 3-2 through 3-6 present each submodel in greater detail, illustrating relevent factors and logical relationships. These submodels are briefly described in the following paragraphs. More detailed descriptions and references may be found in a report prepared by another National Research Council committee (NRC, 1985).

Figure 3-7 combines the submodels to provide an overall account of the risk source, exposure, and health effects. The figures themselves are no more than a visual aid, and may be substantially amplified and revised as FSIS brings its full expertise to bear on risk assessment.

Production Submodel

The first major component of the risk model (Figure 3-2) accounts for all risk factors associated with the production of live poultry. The wholesomeness and safety of poultry products depends on the health of the live birds, their feed, and the environment in which they are raised. Thus, management practices and production technologies are critical risk factors. Important production activities include breeding, hatching, feed milling, and poultry health care, each of which may affect microbiological or chemical hazards that reach the consumer.

Methods of live poultry production may affect the wholesomeness of poultry products in several ways. During breeding and hatching, infection may be transmitted through the ovaries, through contaminated eggs in breeder flocks, or as a result of exposure to infectious agents in the hatchery. Infections may also occur during grow-out (Smitherman et al., 1984).

Other factors of concern are related to production facility management. For example, methods of feed storage can promote or prevent mold growth and the production of mycotoxins, e.g., aflatoxin. Water containing infectious agents such as Salmonella also presents hazards (NRC, 1985, p. 128). The condition of the feed provided during the first few days of a bird's life is particularly important, since it effectively establishes gut flora and the chick's ability to fight off future contaminations (Mead and Impey, 1985; Nurmi, 1985; Snoyenbos et al., 1978). The sanitation of the poultry housing facilities and methods of manure and sewage disposal can also have implications for public health.

Studies of Salmonella ecology clearly establish the genetic stock, feed and feed ingredients, and environmental sources as critical points at which hazards from this microorganism may be controlled during

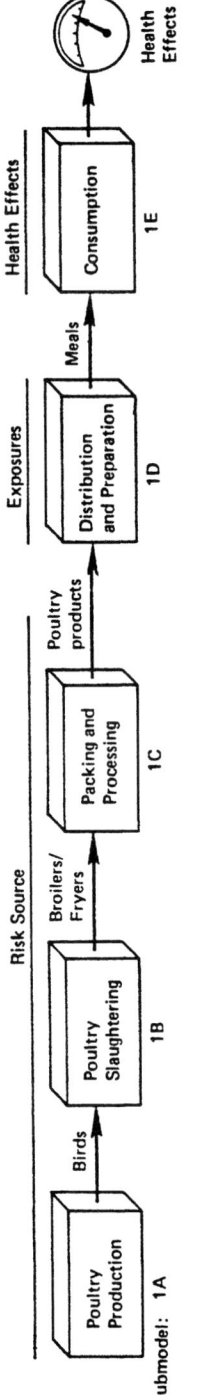

Figure 3-1
Major components (submodels) of the conceptual risk model for poultry production risk assessment.

poultry production (Barnum, 1977; Bryan et al., 1976; NRC, 1969). Despite precautions, however, exposures of poultry to pathogenic microorganisms such as <u>Salmonella</u> are difficult to avoid. Total confinement of primary breeding flocks has been studied as one means for reducing the transmission of <u>Salmonella</u> through eggs. Fumigation techniques have been tried as well. There are methods to reduce the <u>Salmonella</u> contamination of processed feeds; however, feed contamination remains a widespread and serious problem (USDA, 1978).

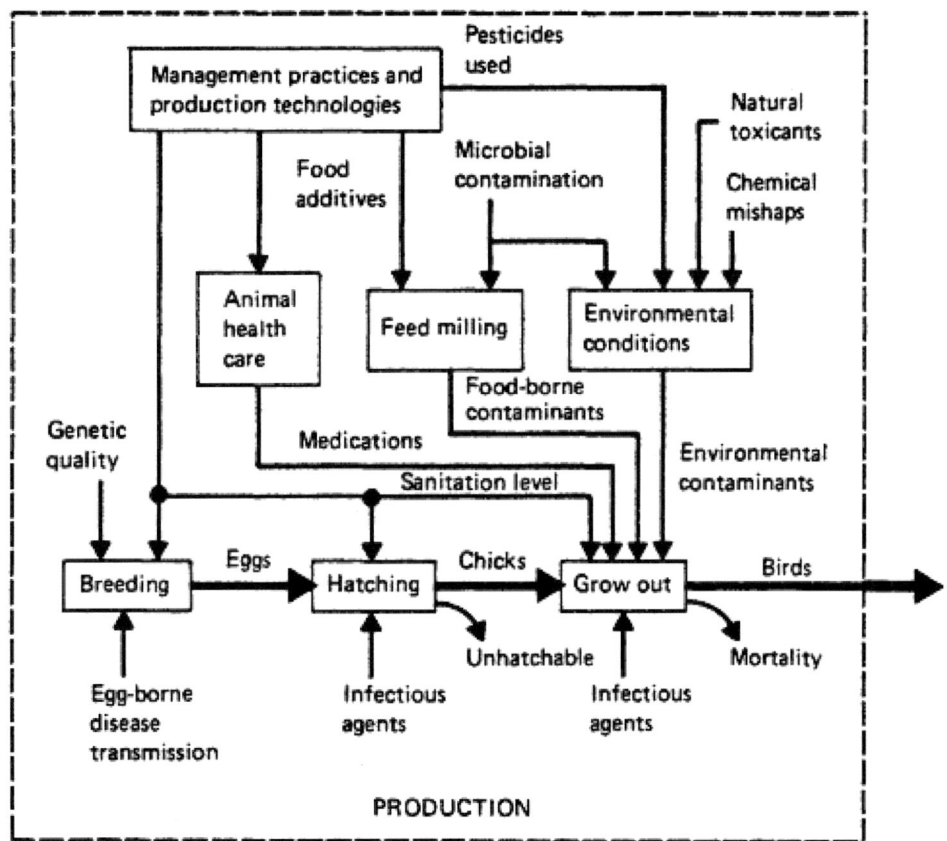

Figure 3-2
Production submodel.

Vaccines administered to prevent economically important diseases may have public health consequences. In addition, most producers rely on a variety of prophylactic medications, especially antimicrobial agents and coccidiostats, to prevent or reduce the prevalence of infectious agents and parasites (North, 1984). The type of antibiotics as well as the quantity and time of their application on farms are critical factors, because the residues from these substances can remain in the tissues and present a health hazard to some people. Residues from drugs and medicated feeds are often found in carcasses when they are administered too soon before slaughter (USDA, 1984a). Drug residues can also result from the accidental mixing of medicated and nonmedicated feeds at the feed mill, during transport to the farm, or at the farm itself. Antibiotic-resistant strains of pathogens may emerge as a result of treating birds or using antibiotics in feed.

Chemical residues can also result if the poultry are exposed to pesticides and other agricultural or industrial chemicals (Booth, 1982; Doull et al., 1980). Pesticides may be applied to animals to control insects or internal parasites, but most exposures of poultry result from the application of pesticides to buildings, crops used for feed, or feed storage areas. Industrial chemicals used in electrical and mechanical equipment, e.g., polychlorinated biphenyls (PCBs) used in some electric power transformers, can also leave residues. If not detected in time, an accident, such as inadvertent contamination with PCB or hexachlorobenzene, could introduce into the food chain high levels of toxic substances that are not normally present (Booth, 1982; Doull et al., 1980).

Thus, poultry production practices have the potential for affecting human health risks by determining whether and the extent to which various hazardous agents enter the poultry supply. They are often responsible for the diseases and contaminants that may be detected during inspection. At present, however, the Food Safety Inspection Service (FSIS) has no responsibility for monitoring the production phase.

Slaughter Submodel

The next major component of the risk model (Figure 3-3) includes the risk factors related to slaughter and the inspection activities conducted during this process. The critical points in slaughtering operations include sanitary conditions during transport and during the slaughtering process itself, as well as antemortem and postmortem inspections and examinations for microbial and chemical contaminants. Live poultry is usually sent by truck to the slaughtering plant in specially built coops, baskets, or batteries. As noted in Chapter 2, antemortem inspection is discretionary and is designed to ensure compliance with regulations, with no apparent mechanism to selectively emphasize those regulations that relate to issues important to the public's health. Nonetheless, most producers include this step in their own quality control programs, in part to provide early data on probable flock condemnation rates.

Poultry raising practices are such that a lot delivered for slaughter tends to have a common genetic and environmental background. In addition, disease incidence in a given lot is likely to be either quite low or fairly high, resulting in distinct lot-to-lot distribution of condemnation rates. However, inspectors conducting antemortem inspection usually have no knowledge of the flock's history to aid them in identifying human health hazards.

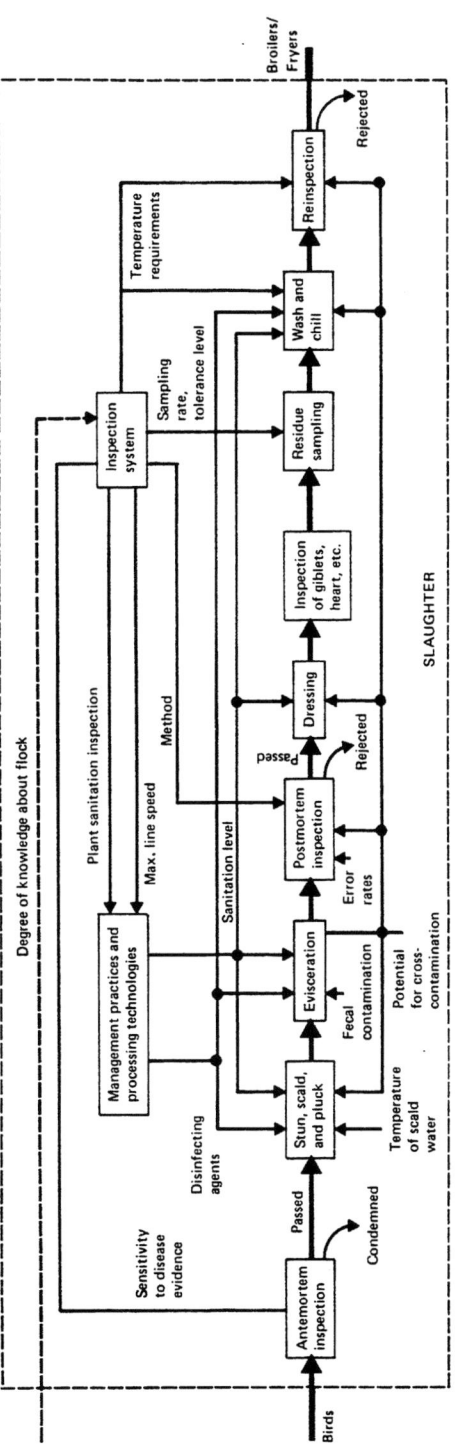

Figure 3-3
Slaughter submodel.

During antemortem inspection, the FSIS inspector has an opportunity to observe birds between the time of arrival and when they are hung on the slaughtering line. Although birds may be rejected as a result of antemortem inspection, the criteria for condemnation are not always sensitive to the hazard posed to human health. For example, a bird developing heat stroke in transit is placed in the same public health category as one in terminal stages of septicemic salmonellosis.

Birds that pass antemortem inspection are placed on a line leading them to the various steps in the slaughtering process and to postmortem inspection. The first step in the slaughtering process is often, but not always, to stun the birds with an electrical shock. Subsequently, the birds pass through steps that may affect human health risk: scalding, the removal of feathers, and the withdrawal of viscera. As in the production phase, the management practices and processing technologies used in these procedures can have a considerable impact on microbial loads.

Most microbial contamination of the poultry's skin surfaces occurs during defeathering (ICMSF, 1980). In one automated study of plant sanitation, Salmonella was isolated more often from pickers (machines provided with many rubber prongs called fingers, which remove all the feathers) than from any of the other equipment sampled, both before and after the start of processing (Campbell et al., 1984). A possible reason for this could be the complex construction of the pickers and the inherent difficulty of adequately cleaning all the picker fingers. The temperature of scald water (52°C; 126°F) and the thorough washing of poultry carcasses are critical in poultry slaughtering operations because of the potential for transfer and cross-contamination of Salmonella and other microorganisms during defeathering (Green et al., 1982).

Perhaps the most important step of sanitary dressing is the proper removal of the gastrointestinal (GI) tract. Since Salmonella and other enteric bacteria originate in the digestive tract and fecal material of the slaughtered bird, it is extremely important to prevent contamination of the carcass by spilled GI tract contents or smeared fecal matter (ICMSF, 1980). The likelihood of contamination increases in birds with localized or generalized diseases, infections, or contamination.

After postmortem inspection, as noted in Chapter 2, the birds are passed as food or condemned in 1 of the 11 categories listed in Table 2-2 . In fiscal year 1983, for all classes of poultry, less than 1% of the poultry examined were condemned during postmortem inspection (USDA, 1984c). In general, inspectors base their condemnation decisions on five criteria: condition of tissue (diseased or abnormal), type of disease (localized or generalized; acute or chronic), impairment of important body functions (e.g., uremia, icterus, toxemia), injurious to health of consumer (e.g., tissues containing toxic chemical residues or infectious agents), and appearance (offensive or repugnant) (USDA, 1984b). Carcasses are usually condemned because of the presence of a visible anatomic lesion or specific condition (e.g., air sacculitis) rather than by cause (e.g., a specific infectious agent). The inspection system is not designed to detect human pathogens unless they produce an observable lesion. Neither pathogenic microorganisms that typically reside in the gastrointestinal tracts and on external surfaces of poultry nor chemical residues are generally detectable by routine organoleptic inspection procedures (i.e., sight, smell, or touch). Condemned carcasses and parts are promptly destroyed to prevent their entrance into the human food chain (Libby and Humphreys, 1975).

Information collected by the U.S. Department of Agriculture in previous years indicates "passed-bird error rates" (percentage of passed birds with gross and visible lesions) of approximately 1% to 1.5% and that there are large inspector-to-inspector and day-to-day variations but small plant-to-plant variations. These estimates were obtained from 1969 to 1973, when condemnation rates were approximately 5%, and are not likely to be applicable now, when condemnation rates are roughly 1% (Booz-Allen & Hamilton, Inc., 1977). They indicate, nevertheless, that error rates may equal a substantial fraction of condemnation rates. Carcasses contaminated with chemical residues and bacteria are generally not identifiable during inspection because these conditions are rarely visible. Therefore, these factors are not included in the error rate.

Other aspects of the inspection process with public health significance are inspection of plant sanitation (Kauffman and Schaffner, 1974), monitoring of residues, and reinspection of carcasses (see Chapter 2).

The residue monitoring program emphasizes the control of chlorinated hydrocarbon pesticides; however, evidence of a variety of other chemicals is also sought. During fiscal year 1983, 424 samples of young chickens were analyzed for 15 different chlorinated hydrocarbon residues. There were 73 positives, but only one that exceeded established tolerances (for chlordane) (USDA, 1986). Some poultry producers operate their own residue programs, working with FSIS to detect violative residues and remove contaminated products from food channels.

Chilling and freezing of poultry carcasses (broilers; fryers) at temperatures of 40°F (4°C) or less within 4 hours after slaughter are critical factors in inhibiting microbial growth (CFR, 1983). Carcass reinspection involves the sampling of carcasses that have passed routine postmortem inspection, dressing, and wash-and-chilling operations (see Chapter 2). Final carcass washing is a risk factor influencing biological contamination levels. Germicides such as chlorine may be helpful, although the efficacy of chlorination under some conditions is not certain (NRC, 1985). The design of final washers used on poultry evisceration lines (e.g., water pressure, nozzle type, location, and procedures) can also influence microbial counts.

Packing and Further Processing Submodel

Packing and further processing of broilers and fryers are also critical factors (Figure 3-4). When carcasses are cut, pathogens on the surfaces of the carcasses, including species of <u>Salmonella, Campylobacter, Clostridium</u>, and <u>Staphylococcus</u>, can contaminate workers' hands, cutting boards, knives, tabletops, saws, and other pieces of equipment, and can then be transferred directly or via cleaning cloths to other equipment. The effectiveness and extent of efforts to minimize cross-contamination at this stage and to improve the sanitation of processing equipment constitute risk factors. The temperature in rooms for deboning, slicing, and storage and the durations of storage are also critical points that determine whether contaminating organisms multiply.

For frozen products the critical points up to the time of freezing are the same as those for chilled products. In addition, proper packaging, rapid freezing, and the time and temperature at which products are frozen and subsequently thawed also influence the counts of microorganisms (Peterson and Gunnerson, 1974). For vacuum-packed poultry products, it is important to maintain anaerobic conditions in a carbon dioxide and nitrogen atmosphere so that growth of the aerobic flora that commonly spoil unpackaged raw poultry can be inhibited.

For dried poultry, the moisture content should be lowered enough to provide shelf stability. It is therefore essential that the drying rapidly decrease the A_w[1] of these products to levels at which pathogens do not multiply. During the drying process, therefore, the rapidity of the procedure and temperature control are critical points. For cooked, uncured products, the quality of the raw ingredients is a critical control point as are the duration of cooking (which should be sufficient to kill yeasts, molds, parasites, and viruses), the temperature of cooking (130-167°F, or 54-75°C), the rate of cooling (pathogens can multiply in cooked products held too long at certain temperatures), the handling of the products after cooking (e.g., an entry point for <u>Salmonella</u>) (Bryan, 1980), equipment sanitation, and subsequent cold storage (when micrococci, streptococci, and other psychrophilic bacteria may multiply). For uncured canned products, acidity is important. Products with a pH of 4.6 or less are considered high-acid products and need only heating to ensure shelf stability. Low-acid uncured canned foods (pH greater than 4.6) must be given time-temperature exposures that kill up to 10^{12} <u>Clostridium botulinum spores. For cured canned poultry, critical factors are proper curing (including adequate salt and nitrite concentrations), quality of</u>

---

[1] A_w (water activity) is the ratio of the water pressure of a food to that of pure water at the same temperature. It is the measure of water in food available for use by microorganisms that have specific cardinal requirements for A_w.

ingredients (with reference to microbes), level of spore contamination, drying process (proper A_w), container integrity, and proper cold storage. The pathogens of most concern in high A_w cured meats are Salmonella, Staphylococcus, and C. botulinum (Ito, 1974; Sebald and Jouglard, 1977).

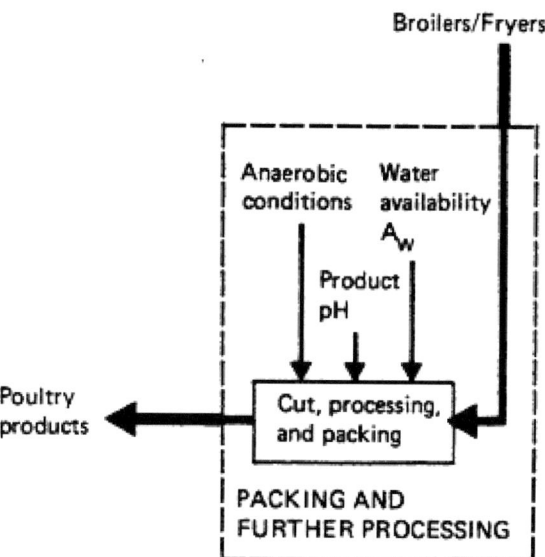

Figure 3-4
Packing and further processing submodel.

The addition of chemicals during processing of poultry is another critical factor. Violative amounts (amounts added above the set tolerance levels) could result in adverse health effects. There are aproximately 1,800 food additives, most of which are flavors and antioxidants. Probably 1% of these are used in poultry products specifically (Joint FAO/WHO Expert Committee on Food Additives, 1983). Other factors with public health implications are concentrations of chlorine used to reduce microbiological contamination (Cantor, 1982; Mead et al., 1975; Zoeteman et al., 1982); toxic compounds (e.g., polycyclic hydrocarbons) produced as a result of heating fresh, smoked, grilled, and cured meats (Meyer, 1960); bone and metal fragments that enter poultry during processing; leaching of chemicals from the packaging material into the food product (e.g., polyvinyl chloride, acrylonitrile) (Karel and Heidelbaugh, 1975; Sacharow, 1979); and the intrinsic chemical (e.g., polymerization, free-radical formation) and physical (e.g., consistency, texture, color) changes that occur in tissues during improper storage (Ames, 1983; Lee, 1983; Roberts, 1981).

Distribution and Preparation Submodel

After processing, microorganisms in poultry products can multiply, spread, and perhaps cross-contaminate other foods unless the products are handled properly in the plant, during transport, in retail outlets, and by the consumer after purchase. Critical risk factors during distribution are the microbial load at the time of shipment, the internal temperature at the time of loading, and the air temperature and movement in the transport vehicle and storage warehouse (Figure 3-5). Insect and rodent control may also be critical during storage of paper-and plastic-packaged dry products. In retail stores, walk-in refrigerators and display cases and cleanliness of cutting boards and blocks, grinders, saws, tenderizers, and cutting utensils are key control points.

The critical factors during preparation in food service establishments and in homes are generally beyond FSIS control, but vary with the product, equipment, and food-service system. The major opportunities for outbreaks of food-borne diseases in both food-service establishments (Bobeng and David, 1977; Bryan, 1981a,b; Bryan and McKinley, 1974; Unklesbay et al., 1977) and homes (Zottola and Wolf, 1980) are presented when cooked foods are held at or near room temperature, when cooked foods are stored in large containers during refrigerated storage, when food is prepared a day or more before serving (Bryan, 1978, 1980), and in any type of food processing plant (Bauman, 1974; DHEW, 1972; Ito, 1974; Kauffman and Schaffner, 1974; Peterson and Gunnerson, 1974; WHO/ICMSF, 1982). Other frequently identified contributory factors are inadequate cooking, inadequate reheating, contamination by infected persons, and cross-contamination by inadequately cleaned equipment (e.g., cutting boards, knives, slicers, grinders, tabletops, and storage pans). Several precautions that can be taken to help avoid these hazards are washing hands after handling raw poultry or when returning to work stations; preventing cross-contamination by thoroughly cleaning utensils, equipment, tabletops, sponges, and cleaning cloths; cooking poultry thoroughly; avoidance of holding cooked poultry at room temperature for long periods; cooling rapidly in shallow containers any leftovers or food prepared for consumption on subsequent days; and reheating leftovers thoroughly. Programs designed to provide information on such matters as Hazard Analysis Critical Control Point principles, poultry science, food microbiology, and safe food handling operations will all help in reducing exposure levels.

Health Effects (Consumption) Submodel

Enteric bacterial agents are primarily health hazards for the consuming public. Less commonly, they are occupational hazards in the meat packing industry. The major agents are <u>Salmonella</u>, <u>Campylobacter</u>, and <u>Clostridium perfringens</u> (Bryan, 1980). Each year as many as 2 million Americans are affected by salmonellosis —an important health effect that is clearly linked to poultry (Figure 3-6) (USDA, 1978); however, only a fraction of these cases are ever reported. Antimicrobial-resistant salmonellae account for a steadily increasing number of salmonellosis cases in the United States and can be traced to food animals, including poultry (Holmberg and Blake, 1984). This

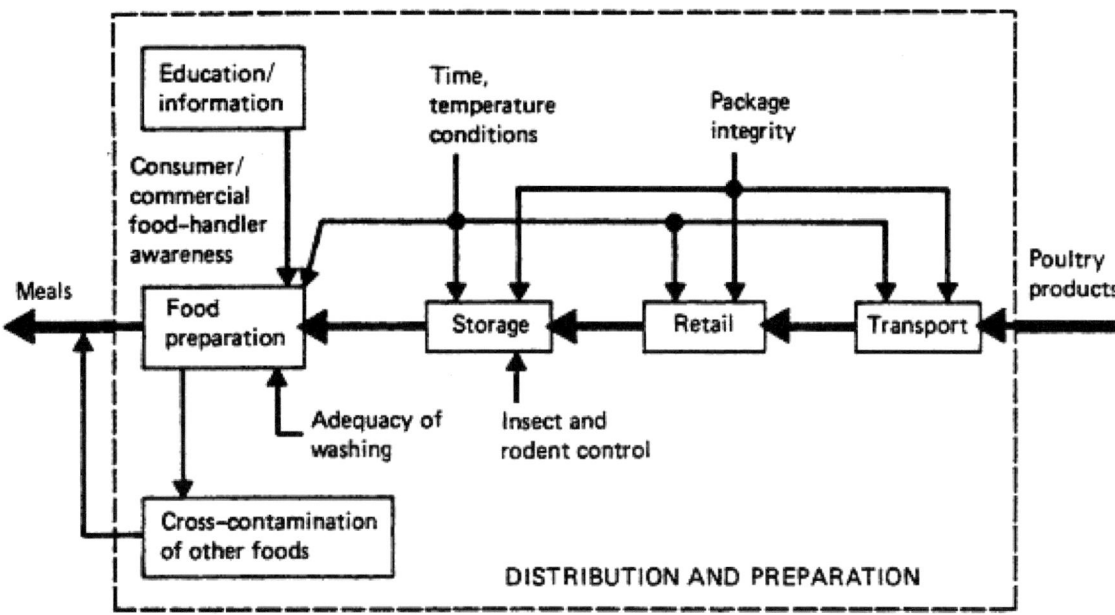

Figure 3-5
Distribution and preparation submodel.

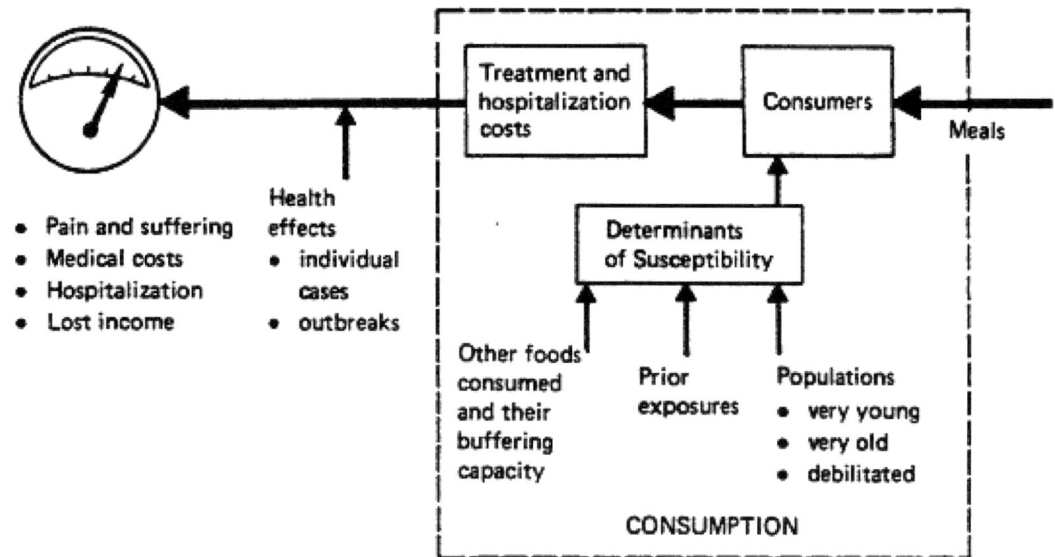

Figure 3-6
Consumption submodel.

disease accounts for much pain and suffering and is costly in terms of medical care, hospitalization, and lost income through absence from work.

Campylobacter presents a somewhat similar health problem. Although this microorganism tends not to multiply in food at room temperatures (Skirrow, 1982), it can survive on chilled carcasses for months (Oosterom et al., 1983). Since antemortem and postmortem inspection can rarely identify Campylobacter or Clostridium perfringens (CDC, 1983) in infected poultry, prevention of carcass contamination by fecal matter is a critical control point, as it is for salmonellae.

Toxic chemicals, including carcinogens, may also contribute to adverse health effects in humans. For example, polycyclic aromatic hydrocarbons (PAHs) are commonly found in fresh, smoked, grilled, and cured poultry (NRC, 1985). Of the more than 100 PAH compounds identified, 5 are known carcinogens when given orally, and 3 of these 5 are part of the average U.S. diet. The impact of these compounds on humans at ordinary dietary levels throughout a lifetime is not known (Meyer, 1960).

USE OF THE RISK MODEL

The risk model described above accounts for all major elements involved in bringing poultry products to the consumer and some specific factors that may influence the safety and wholesomeness of the products and the consequent health impacts on consumers (Figure 3-7). The model provides a basis for risk assessment in that it serves as a logical road map that can be used in the evaluation of current or proposed strategies for reducing and controlling risks. The method of assessment consists of evaluating the extent to which the control strategy affects each critical control point and then determining the implications of these effects. To the extent that quantitative data exist, a well-defined, quantitative measure of risk may be determined through application of logic inherent in the risk model. In the absence of such data, qualitative judgments may still be used to develop a logical and rigorous evaluation of alternative strategies.

The risk model also suggests a generalized logic for investigating and comparing alternative strategies for controlling human health risks. Specifically, evaluation of the relative effectiveness of alternative controls for a specific risk requires the following steps:

1. Assess the magnitude of the health risk of concern. For example, how serious is the risk of ingesting microbial contaminants in poultry?
2. Review the risk model to determine its adequacy for the intended purpose, and use it to identify and organize the critical factors that determine or influence the magnitude of

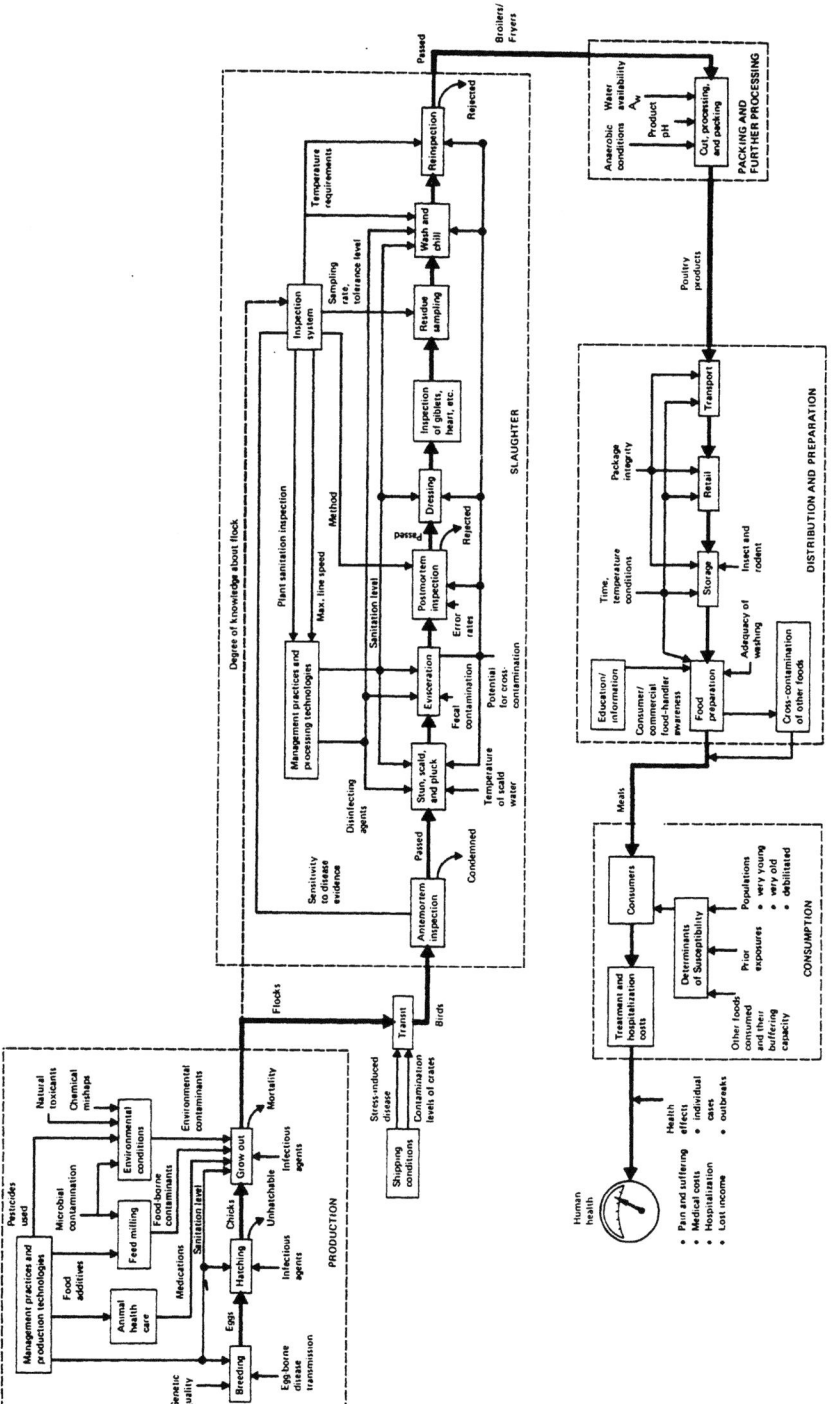

Figure 3-7
The conceptual risk model for assessment of human health risks associated with poultry.

the risk. For example, the number and severity of potential health effects may be influenced by the level of microbial contamination of feed, the degree of contamination of the carcass during evisceration, the extent of cross-contamination during cutting, and other factors.

3. Compare the degree to which alternative strategies can affect the critical factors.
4. Use the conceptual risk model to determine how impacts on critical factors relate to incremental changes in the likelihood that health effects will occur in consumers and the magnitude of those effects.

Data are currently insufficient to permit the last step to be based on formal quantitative models. Nevertheless, this task can be performed qualitatively by using the risk model to guide the professional judgments necessary to reach a qualitative conclusion about the impacts on human health. As appropriate quantitative data are collected, the various steps outlined above may be used to produce quantitative measures of risk. Regardless of whether risk estimates are quantitative or qualitative, such assessments are essential to the identification and selection of FSIS strategies for protecting public health. Described below is a generalized logic for incorporating risk assessment into the planning process.

USING RISK ASSESSMENTS TO PROTECT HEALTH

A substantial assurance that health risks do not reach unacceptable levels is surely a critical function of the FSIS program. Potential adverse health consequences vary in frequency and severity, and evidence concerning them ranges from nearly nothing to conclusive. An optimal health-protection program (including inspection) can exploit these variations both to increase effectiveness of inspection procedures and to reduce costs of their implementation. Put simply, it is important to determine what types of risk and evidence pertaining to that risk justifies what set of actions.

Limited information and uncertainties create difficulties in each step of risk assessment. Hazard identification is often uncertain; e.g., there may be only poor evidence on the clinical significance of certain strains of Salmonella found in broiler chickens or on the carcinogenicity of a chemical residue. Dose-response relationships are hard to establish with precision and may vary from time to time, place to place, and (especially) consumer to consumer. It is also difficult to assess exposures with any degree of completeness or certainty, since only a small percentage of broiler chickens can be tested for specific chemical or microbial hazards. Because of these and countless similar problems, knowledge about the health risks attributable to broiler chickens is somewhat fragmentary and uncertain.

The current FSIS inspection program is relatively inflexible and is noe well suited for providing information needed to resolve these uncertainties. For example, every bird must pass organoleptic inspection, and line speeds are fixed at specific rates. Sample sizes for testing and surveillance of chemical residues are also fixed; no opportunity is provided for adjusting the detection sensitivity to changing perceptions regarding the magnitudes of the hazards or the likelihood that residues will be found. Opportunities for resolving uncertainties are missed; for example, birds condemned during organoleptic inspection are not examined to learn what they can teach regarding the assessment and abatement of health risks. The inspection itself cannot ordinarily distinguish contaminated from uncontaminated birds, whether the contamination is microbial or chemical.

Information might be collected to build a base of knowledge for improving inspection effectiveness. For example, if the first, approximately random 10% of a flock is unusually healthy, the remaining 90% is likely to be healthy too. An infection in one grow-out house may well be present in an adjacent house. If a prohibited practice is detected at one place or time in a slaughter operation, it is possible that there maybe other prohibited practices at other places and times in that operation. Indeed, inspectors often believe quite strongly that they can distinguish good flocks and good operators from bad ones.

This continuum in knowledge and the parallel continuum in risk are not, on the whole, reflected in either the strategies of FSIS for inspection or the more general control of health hazards. The methods used cannot be tailored to changing situations and do not maximize the potential for learning. Thus, an opportunity exists to improve both the public health and the cost-effectiveness of the FSIS inspection procedures by adopting procedures capable of accounting for substantial gradations in both risk and knowledge about risks in general and about circumstances contributing to risk. To protect health, inspection should be deliberately and objectively targeted to maximize, for a given expenditure of resources, the return in reduced morbidity and mortality. This return will vary from one activity to another, from one producer to another, from one time to another, and in other ways.

Formal risk assessment is the key to capturing, organizing, and interpreting the evidence that can be brought to bear on the optimum use of inspection resources. It will identify problems in a clear and organized way; produce the best possible estimate of the likelihood that a risk exists, and if so, its size; and make clear the kinds and degrees of uncertainty attached to that estimate. This information can then be translated into a detailed strategy to protect human health, including the development of specific regulations and instructions to inspection staff.

A comprehensive strategy for reducing the health risks attributable to poultry should be based on a broad conceptual model of how those risks arise and on assessments of the nature and magnitude of those risks made at the highest level of precision attainable. Furthermore: the risk reduction strategy should be cost effective and designed to take advantage of the full range of tools available to FSIS. Any health protection program is likely to involve several steps, but there is no agreed-upon classification of these steps, such as there is for the four steps in risk assessment. Some of these activities are listed below. Their order should not be construed as an implication of their priority.

- Establish objectives and set priorities.
- Identify and analyze alternatives for achieving priority objectives such as the following: e.g., 100% organoleptic inspection or a requirement for a withdrawal period after use of a drug.
- Identify potential hazards and set tolerances or action levels (targets and goals) for each, including considerations of possible synergistic interactions.
- Select and implement a control program.
- Conduct monitoring and surveillance and interpret results.
- Take appropriate steps to ensure compliance (by producers) and enforcement (by FSIS).
- Conduct research to improve the model, the risk assessments, or the data on which they are based.

These kinds of activities should be developed as an integrated package; they are substantially less independent than the steps in risk assessment. Several catagories of such activities are discussed below.

Establish Priorities

Any feasible program for risk management will require establishment of priorities for reducing or eliminating factors that contribute to risk. Such priorities and the frequency and intensity of monitoring should be based on risk assessment, but for most kinds of FSIS interventions it is only the relative risks of the various alternatives that are of concern. For example, in choosing among postmortem inspection strategies, it is the potential increase or decrease from current levels of health risks that is most important.

Thus, there would be much value in having a scheme for relative ranking of all poultry-borne risks, including microbial hazards, even if the absolute magnitudes of those risks remain uncertain. In Chapter 5 , for example, it is shown how different carcinogenic hazards can be ranked on a common qualitative scale. A broader system of ranking may require a substantial research program as well as field testing.

A scheme for assessing relative risks need not include estimation of the absolute risk of any of the substances to be ranked. It is necessary only that the scheme incorporate in a systematic way some measures of both pathogenicity and exposure. Both of these components are essential and must be determined to an adequate degree of accuracy. For example, the data on Class 1, 2, and 3 chemicals (see Chapter 5) vary widely in quality and content, and these differences must be taken into account in a systematic way.

The primary purpose of a relative risk assessment is to ensure that two major risk-management activities—monitoring of feed and water and monitoring of poultry products (including whole birds)—are given a level of emphasis reflecting the probability that the risk factor will be found in food intended for human consumption, the level of risk that may result if it escapes detection, and the extent to which the risk can be reduced.

Identify Problems of Risk Management, and Set Acceptable Levels of Risk

After analyzing a broad range of hazards, Lowrance (1976) concluded that "a thing is safe if its risks are judged acceptable." This is not a tautology; perfect safety is a chimera, but very small risks may be deemed acceptable when the costs (in the broadest sense) of their further reduction exceed the expected benefits. For example, FDA does not in general concern itself with carcinogens that are believed to produce cancer risks of less than one per million persons exposed at the maximum allowable dose over a lifetime. Acceptability of risk depends on many things, including the type of outcome (e.g., skin rash vs. cancer), whether the risk is already common or familiar, and whether the risk is known to exposed persons and assumed voluntarily (Fischhoff et al., 1978). Perceptions of risk to health are important whether or not they are in line with the best quantitative estimates.

Both the definition of risk and the determination that certain risks cannot be eliminated at an acceptable cost are generally very difficult. Risk management, including the setting of acceptable levels of risk, is a political rather than scientific task and hence outside the committee's purview. The committee notes, however, that risk management should ordinarily be based on the best available scientific risk assessment and an objective analysis of the appropriate role of risk assessment in risk management. Furthermore, risk-management goals should be precisely stated in quantitative, evaluable terms. For example, a maximum tolerance level below the lowest detectable level (microbial or chemical) would be unenforceable.

Monitoring and Surveillance

There will be a continuing need for monitoring and surveillance to ensure that FSIS program goals are met—goals that can be partitioned into structure, process, and outcome. It will also be necessary to fine-tune inspection activities and to update the system to keep pace with changing risks and production practices.

Of particular importance for the monitoring program is the selection of sampling rates. Statistical sampling strategies can be devised to ensure, with a specified degree of confidence, that products containing excessive levels of chemical residues are identified for removal from the food supply. The desirable degree of confidence for potentially high risk substances should be greater than for other substances. In Chapter 5 of this report, the committee recommends specific criteria for chemical residues posing different levels of potential risk to public health. Chapter 6 describes a risk ranking scheme, which can be used not only to develop monitoring strategies, but also to aid other data gathering efforts.

Risk assessment plays several important roles in a program to control or eliminate health hazards posed by broiler chickens. All are based on applying, with varying degrees of rigor, the elements of a conceptual model of risk and rely on the use of specific types of data. An effective risk management scheme will require each of these program elements, although not all need to be within the direct control of FSIS (indeed, some are already established at FDA and EPA). Nevertheless, it is important that FSIS ensure adequate coverage of the full range of activities needed in risk management and that the agency acquire substantial knowledge of the adequacy of each activity.

REFERENCES

Ames, B. N. 1983. Dietary carcinogens and anticarcinogens: Oxygen radicals and degenerative diseases. Science 221:1256-1264.

Barnum, D. A., ed. 1977. Proceedings of the International Symposium on Salmonella and Prospects for Control held at the University of Guelph, June 8-11, 1977. University of Guelph, Guelph, Ontario, Canada. 200 pp.

Bauman, H. E. 1974. The HACCP concept and microbiological hazard categories. Food Technol. 28:30, 32, 34, 74.

Bobeng, B. J., and B. D. David. 1977. HACCP models for quality control of entree production in food service systems. J. Food Protect. 40:632-638.

Booth, N. H. 1982. Drug and chemical residues in the edible tissues of animals. Pp. 1065-1113 in N. H. Booth and L. E. McDonald, eds. Veterinary Pharmacology and Therapeutics, 5th ed. Iowa State University Press, Ames, Iowa.

Booz-Allen & Hamilton, Inc. 1977. Study of the Federal Meat and Poultry Inspection System, Vol. II—Opportunities for Change—An Evaluation of Specific Alternatives. Prepared for the U.S. Department of Agriculture. Contract No. 53-3142-6-3614. U.S. Department of Agriculture, Washington, D.C. 351 pp.

Bryan, F. L. 1978. Factors that contribute to outbreaks of foodborne disease. J. Food Protect. 41:816-827.

Bryan, F. L. 1980. Foodborne diseases in the United States associated with meat and poultry . 3. Food Protect. 43:140-150.

Bryan, F. L. 1981a. Hazard analysis critical control point approach: Epidemiologic rationale and application to food service operations. J. Environ. Health 44:7-14.

Bryan, F. L. 1981b. Hazard analysis of food service operations. Food Technol. 35:78-87.

Bryan, F. L., and T. W. McKinley. 1974. Prevention of foodborne illness by time-temperature control of thawing, cooking, chilling and reheating turkeys in school lunch kitchens. J. Milk Food Technol. 37:420-429.

Bryan, F. L., H. Anderson, R. K. Anderson, K. J. Baker, H. Matsuura, T. W. McKinley, R. Swanson, and E. Todd. 1976. Procedures to Investigate Food-borne Illness, 3rd ed. International Association of Milk, Food and Environmental Sanitarians, Ames, Iowa. 74 pp.

Campbell, D. F., R. W. Johnston, M. W. Wheeler, K. V. Nagaraja, C. D. Szymansaki, and B. S. Pomeroy. 1984. Effects of the evisceration and cooling processes on the incidence of Salmonella in fresh dressed turkeys grown under Salmonella-controlled and uncontrolled environments. Poult. Sci. 63:1069-1072.

Cantor, K. P. 1982. Epidemiological evidence of carcinogenicity of chlorinated organics in drinking water. Environ. Health Perspect. 26:187-195.

CDC (Centers for Disease Control). 1983. Foodborne Disease Surveillance, Annual Summary 1981. HHS Publ. No. (CDC) 83-8185. Centers for Disease Control, Public Health Service, U.S. Department of Health and Human Services, Atlanta. 41 pp.

CFR (Code of Federal Regulations). 1983. Title 9, Animals and Animal Products; Section 381.66, Temperatures and chilling and freezing procedures. U.S. Government Printing Office, Washington, D.C.

DHEW (U.S. Department of Health, Education, and Welfare). 1972. Proceedings of the 1971 National Conference on Food Protection held in Denver, Colorado, April 4-8, 1971. Sponsored by American Public Health Association. DHEW Publ. No. (FDA) 72-2015. U.S. Food and Drug Administration, U.S. Department of Health, Education, and Welfare, Washington, D.C. 242 pp.

Doull, J., C. D. Klaassen, and M. O. Amdur, eds. 1980. Casarett and Doull's Toxicology—The Basic Science of Poisons, 2nd ed. Macmillan, New York. 778 pp.

Fischhoff, B., P. Slovic, S. Lichtenstein, S. Read, and B. Combs. 1978. How safe is safe enough? A psychometric study of attitudes towards technological risks and benefits. Policy Sci. 9:127-152.

Green, S. S., A. B. Moran, R. W. Johnston, P. Uhler, and J. Chiu. 1982. The incidence of Salmonella species and serotypes in young whole chicken carcasses in 1979 as compared with 1967. Poult. Sci. 61:288-293.

Holmberg, S. D., and P. A. Blake. 1984. Staphylococcal food poisoning in the United States: New facts and old misconceptions. J. Am. Med. Assoc. 251:487-489.

ICMSF (International Commission on Microbiological Specifications for Foods). 1980. Microbial Ecology of Foods, Vol. II: Food Commodities. Academic Press, New York. 664 pp.

Ito, K. 1974. Microbiological critical control points in canned foods. Food Technol. 28:46, 48.

Joint FAO/WHO Expert Committee on Food Additives. 1983. Evaluation of Certain Food Additives and Contaminants. 27th Report of the Joint FAO/WHO Expert Committee on Food Additives, Technical Report Series No. 696. World Health Organization, Geneva. 47 pp.

Karel, M., and N. D. Heidelbaugh. 1975. Effects of packaging on nutrients. Pp. 412-462 in R. S. Harris and E. Karmas, eds. Nutritional Evaluation of Food Processing , 2nd ed. AVI Publishing, Westport, Conn.

Kauffman, F. L., and R. M. Schaffner. 1974. Hazard analysis, critical control points and good manufacturing practices regulations (sanitation) in food plant inspections. Pp. 402-407 in the Proceedings of the IV International Congress on Food Science and Technology held in Madrid, Spain, September 22-27, 1974. Instituto de Agroquimicay Technologia de Alimentos, Valencia, Spain.

Lee, F. A. 1983. Basic Food Chemistry, 2nd ed. AVI Publishing, Westport, Conn. 564 pp.

Libby, J. A., and M. R. Humphreys. 1975. Post-mortem dispositions. Pp. 85-186 in J. A. Libby, ed. Meat Hygiene, 4th ed. Lea & Febiger, Philadelphia.

Lowrance, W. W. 1976. Of Acceptable Risk. Science and the Determination of Safety. William Kaufmann, Los Altos, Calif. 180 pp.

Mead, G. C., and C. S. Impey. 1985. Control of Salmonella colonization in poultry flocks by defined gut-flora treatment. Pp. 72-79 in G. H. Snoyenbos, ed. Proceedings of the International Symposium on Salmonella held in New Orleans, Louisiana, July 19-20, 1984. American Association of Avian Pathologists, Kennett Square, Pa.

Mead, G. C., B. W. Adams, and R. T. Parry. 1975. The effectiveness of in-plant chlorination in poultry processing. Br. Poult. Sci. 16:517-526.

Meyer, L. H., ed. 1960. Food Chemistry. Reinhold Organic Chemistry and Biochemistry Textbook Series. Reinhold, New York. 385 pp.

North, M. O. 1984. Commercial Chicken Production Manual, 3rd ed. Animal Science Textbook Series. AVI Publishing, Westport, Conn. 714 pp.

NRC (National Research Council). 1969. An Evaluation of the Salmonella Problem. Report of the Committee on Salmonella, Division of Biology and Agriculture. National Academy of Sciences, Washington, D.C. 207 pp.

NRC (National Research Council). 1983. Risk Assessment in the Federal Government: Managing the Process. Report of the Committee on the Institutional Means for Assessment of Risks to Public Health, Commission on Life Sciences. National Academy Press, Washington, D.C. 203 pp.

NRC (National Research Council). 1985. Meat and Poultry Inspection: The Scientific Basis of the Nation's Program. Report of the Committee on the Scientific Basis of the Nation's Meat and Poultry Inspection Program, Food and Nutrition Board. National Academy Press, Washington, D.C. 209 pp.

Nurmi, E. 1985. Use of competitive exclusion in prevention of salmonellae and other enteropathogenic bacteria infections in poultry. Pp. 64-71 in G. H. Snoyenbos, ed. Proceedings of the International Symposium on Salmonella held in New Orleans, Louisiana, July 19-20, 1984. American Association of Avian Pathologists, Kennett Square, Pa.

Oosterom, J., G. J. A. De Wilde, E. De Boer, L. H. De Blaauw, and H. Karman. 1983. Survival of Campylobacter jejuni during poultry processing and pig slaughtering. J. Food Protect. 46:702-706.

Peterson, A. C., and R. E. Gunnerson. 1974. Microbiological critical control points in frozen foods. Food Technol. 28:37-44.

Roberts, H. R., ed. 1981. Food Safety. Wiley, New York. 339 pp.

Sacharow, S. 1979. Packaging Regulations. AVI Publishing, Westport, Conn. 207 pp.

Sebald, M., and J. Jouglard. 1977. Aspects actuels du botulisme. Rev. Prat. 27:173-176.

Skirrow, M. B. 1982. Campylobacter enteritis—The first 5 years. J. Hyg. 89:175-184.

Smitherman, R. E., C. A. Genigeorgis, and T. B. Farver. 1984. Preliminary observations on the occurrence of Campylobacter jejuni at four California chicken ranches. J. Food Protect. 47:293-298.

Snoyenbos, G. H., O. M. Weinack, and C. F. Smyser. 1978. Protecting chicks and poults from salmonellae by oral administration of "normal gut microflora." Avian Dis. 22:273-287.

Unklesbay, N. F., R. B. Maxcy, M. E. Knickrehm, K. E. Stevenson, M. L. Cremer, and M. E. Mathews. 1977. Food service systems: Product flow and microbial quality and safety of foods. Research Bulletin 1018. College of Agriculture, Agriculture Experiment Station, University of Missouri, Columbia, Mo. 36 pp.

USDA (U.S. Department of Agriculture). 1978. Recommendations for Reduction and Control of Salmonellosis. Report of the U.S. Advisory Committee on Salmonella. Food Safety and Quality Service, U.S. Department of Agriculture, Washington, D.C. 30 pp.

USDA (U.S. Department of Agriculture). 1984a. FSIS Facts: The National Residue Program. FSIS-18. Food Safety and Inspection Service, U.S. Department of Agriculture , Washington, D.C. 4 pp.

USDA (U.S. Department of Agriculture). 1984b. Livestock Carcass Disposition Review. Program Training Division, Meat and Poultry Inspection Technical Services, Food Safety and Inspection Service, U.S. Department of Agriculture, Denton, Tex. 74 pp.

USDA (U.S. Department of Agriculture). 1984c. Statistical Summary: Federal Meat and Poultry Inspection for Fiscal Year 1983. FSIS-14. Food Safety and Inspection Service, U.S. Department of Agriculture, Washington, D.C. 34 pp.

USDA (U.S. Department of Agriculture). 1986. Domestic Residue Data Book: National Residue Program 1983. Science Program, Food Safety and Inspection Service, U.S. Department of Agriculture, Washington, D.C. 95 pp.

WHO/ICMSF (World Health Organization/International Commission on Microbiological Specifications for Foods). 1982. Report of the WHO/ICMSF Meeting on Hazard Analysis: Critical Control Point System in Food Hygiene. World Health Organization, Geneva.

Zoeteman, B. C. J., J. Hrubec, E. de Greef, and H. J. Kool. 1982. Mutagenic activity associated with by-products of drinking water disinfection by chlorine, chlorine dioxide, ozone and UV-irradiation. Environ. Health Perspect. 46:197-205.

Zottola, E. A., and I. D. Wolf. 1980. Recipe hazard analysis—RHAS—a systematic approach to analyzing potential hazards in a recipe for food preparation-preservation. J. Food Protect. 44:560-564.

Chapter 4

Application of the Model to Microbiological Hazards

In the report <u>Meat and Poultry Inspection</u>, published in 1985, a National Research Council committee stated that <u>Salmonella</u> spp. and <u>Campylobacter jejuni</u> were the currently recognized major poultry-borne causes of illness in consumers, but that antemortem and postmortem inspection methods in effect at that time were inadequate to detect these organisms (NRC, 1985b). That committee recommended that FSIS intensify its efforts to control and eliminate contamination with microorganisms that cause disease in consumers. Specific recommendations to achieve this goal included education of producers, processors, food handlers, and consumers; determination of etiologic agents responsible for gross lesions resulting in condemnation; development of a trace-back capability to determine where pathogenic microorganisms contaminate the poultry between farm and table; and emphasis on the Hazard Analysis Critical Control Point (HACCP) concept in the inspection process (NRC, 1985b).

This chapter summarizes a method for identifying and describing risks associated with microbiological contamination of chickens and applies these methods to an evaluation of specific pathogens. The committee made no effort to consider the occupational hazards presented by microorganisms in the workplace (i.e., in chicken slaughtering and processing plants), nor did it evaluate all possible pathogens associated with chickens. Rather, this chapter is designed to serve as a model for subsequent refinement, including collection of additional data needed for risk assessment of microorganisms, and to provide a basis for the development of initial risk-management strategies.

METHODOLOGY USED TO DESCRIBE AND IDENTIFY RISKS

Hazard Identification and Evaluation

<u>General Approach</u>. Several basic questions arise in the identification and evaluation of the public health hazard associated with a specific microbial agent. For example, is the microorganism potentially hazardous to health, i.e., is it a pathogen in humans? How does susceptibility vary from person to person or group to group? Are

all microorganisms in this species, class, or other classification equally hazardous? If the microorganism is a hazard, what disease can it cause? With what frequency does this microorganism cause disease?

The question of whether a microorganism is harmful to health has traditionally been approached by linking known disease syndromes with specific microorganisms. The criteria necessary to identify a microorganism as the etiologic agent for a disease were codified in the late 19th century as Koch's postulates' the microorganism must always be found in the diseased animal, but not in healthy ones; the organism must be isolated from diseased animals and grown in pure culture away from the animal; the organism isolated in pure culture must initiate and reproduce the disease when reinoculated into susceptible animals; and the organism should be reisolated from the experimentally infected animals. Although documentation of all four criteria is not always possible for human pathogens because of ethical considerations, Koch's postulates provide a framework for determining whether a microorganism is hazardous to human health.

In considering the potential health hazard of a microorganism, it is necessary to define the population under consideration. A large number of microorganisms are not pathogenic for normal people but can cause disease and death in susceptible hosts, e.g., persons with underlying diseases that compromise their immunocompetence or who have received chemotherapeutic agents that affect their immune response. For patients whose immune response is totally suppressed (such as patients receiving bone marrow transplants), virtually every microorganism is a potential pathogen, making it difficult to distinguish precisely between pathogens and nonpathogens without some notion of the immune status of the target population.

In defining the health hazard caused by a particular microorganism, it is also necessary to understand the organism's virulence factors, or factors that serve as markers for virulence. For many microorganisms, only a small percentage of strains within a species possess a specific plasmid or chromosomally defined factors that permit the organism to cause disease. For example, Escherichia coli is the dominant aerobic bacterium in all normal human stool samples, and most strains of E. coli are harmless to a healthy adult; however, some carry specific virulence plasmids that have been associated with at least four distinct disease syndromes, including toxin-mediated secretory diarrhea and an invasive dysentary syndrome (Levine, 1985). Similarly, only 1% of environmental Vibrio parahaemolyticus strains produce a hemolysin, which is correlated with their ability to cause disease (Morris and Black, 1985). For many microorganisms, we still have only a rudimentary understanding of virulence factors. Further research may help to explain apparently contradictory data regarding the pathogenicity of certain species of microorganisms.

It is also necessary to understand the disease syndrome and related manifestations. Some microorganisms may only cause mild disease, such as the relatively mild diarrhea seen with many nontoxigenic species of Vibrio; other organisms, such as Salmonella, may also be associated with bacteremia, meningitis, other serious morbidity, and death. Host susceptibility may influence the extent of disease caused by a microorganism. For example, Salmonella bacteremia is more likely to be seen in a patient with sickle-cell disease or an underlying malignancy, whereas meningitis occurs most frequently in neonates. Virulence factors may also influence the severity of disease. For example, strains of Vibrio cholerae that lack the gene for cholera toxin production generally cause only mild disease, whereas fully toxigenic strains can cause rapidly progressive dehydration and circulatory collapse in a previously healthy adult.

Finally, one needs to have data on the extent of disease caused by the microorganism (are there 10 cases in the United States per year, or 10,000?) and some index of disease severity, such as the number of hospitalizations or deaths attributable to the microorganism. The overall public health impact of a microorganism that causes a large number of mild cases resulting in few hospitalizations and no deaths may be significantly less than one responsible for only a few cases but with high rates of hospitalization and mortality.

Sources of Data. The extent of the human health hazard presented by certain microorganisms must usually be determined by synthesizing data from a variety of sources, including studies in volunteers, animal models, and epidemiological studies. Approximations of disease incidence can be based on epidemiological data and on numbers of cases and deaths reported through state and national reporting systems.

For ethical reasons, studies in volunteers are generally limited to healthy adults and to agents that cause only mild disease or for which there is good, effective therapy, but they can provide the best data on pathogenicity, permitting direct testing of Koch's postulates. These studies may also be useful in determining the relationship between dose and infection rates, in characterizing the disease syndrome, and, with an appropriate experimental design, in identifying specific virulence factors. However, they generally cannot be used to develop data on the disease in immunocompromised persons or other high-risk hosts.

Many microorganisms are adapted to specific species, so that they cause disease in only one or a few host species. Therefore, animal models cannot always be used to determine whether a specific microorganism will be pathogenic in humans. Once it has been shown that specific disease manifestations in an animal correlate with disease manifestations in humans, e.g., the correlation between the ability of an E. coli strain to cause keratoconjunctivitis in the guinea pig and its ability to invade enterocytes and cause dysentery in humans (Serény, 1955), animal models can be useful in characterizing virulence factors or in identifying markers for virulence.

Epidemiological studies can provide evidence that an organism is pathogenic by fulfilling one or more of Koch's postulates. For example, studies may demonstrate that a certain microorganism is often found among patients with diarrhea but not among controls, suggesting that the microorganism is responsible for the diarrhea. Similarly, a study of disease outbreaks may demonstrate that one microorganism is significantly associated with illness among patients and is present in the food or other product incriminated as the cause of the outbreak. Epidemiological studies also permit characterization of microbial disease syndromes and can provide information on susceptibility and disease manifestations in persons other than normal healthy adults. Long-term follow-up may also be possible in such studies, permitting identification of chronic syndromes that may not be apparent in short-term experiments in volunteers.

Approximations of incidence can be based on information from epidemiological studies and data reported through national reporting systems. For example, the Centers for Disease Control (CDC) collects national surveillance data on diseases caused by many specific microorganisms, including some of the food-borne bacterial pathogens. However, the number of cases reported through these systems is only a fraction of the actual number. Cases are not reported if a patient does not seek medical attention (e.g., when microorganisms cause relatively mild disease), if the doctor does not order appropriate diagnostic tests (such as a stool culture) for patients that are seen, or if the positive test result is not reported to the appropriate health authorities. By using information from outbreak investigations and other epidemiological studies, it may be possible to obtain a very rough estimate of the actual number of cases that occur for each reported case. For example, it has been estimated that only 1 out of every 20 Shigella infections in the United States is reported (Rosenberg et al., 1977), and possibly as few as 1 out of every 100 Salmonella cases (Aserkoff et al., 1970). Rates of hospitalization and mortality (which may be more complete) derived from epidemiological studies can also be used to estimate incidence rates in the community.

Dose-Response Studies

General Approach. For any one person, a certain number of microorganisms is usually necessary to establish an infection; no infection results when fewer microorganisms are present. This threshold value may differ widely from person to person or time to time, depending on such factors as host susceptibility, the method and vehicle with which the inoculum is presented, and the virulence of the microorganism. Nonetheless, it is sometimes possible to estimate the percentage of normal, healthy adults that will become infected after exposure to a viral or bacterial inoculum of known size.

When determining the dose response of infectious agents, one must also consider the rate of asymptomatic or subclinical infection. Not all persons who become infected with a microorganism develop signs and symptoms of disease. Asymptomatic infections may be quite common, and may be dependent on many factors. For example, only one out of every two or three young adults infected with Epstein-Bart virus will develop signs and symptoms of infectious mononucleosis; few children infected with the virus will have any symptoms at all.

Some infectious agents cause disease by producing toxins that may cause an incremental increase in the severity of illness with increasing toxin levels, rather than a threshold response. The botulinal toxin is one example: food-borne botulism is caused by a preformed neurotoxin present in contaminated food, and disease manifestations and severity correlate directly with the amount of toxin consumed.

Sources of Data. Dose-response data on humans are derived primarily from experiments in volunteers. In these studies, the bacterial or vital inoculum can be carefully controlled; however, they are restricted to healthy adults and usually use a defined laboratory strain that may have atypical virulence. Data on the dose response of food-borne pathogens have also been collected in investigations of outbreaks. These are based on estimates of the amount of food consumed and measurements of the concentration of the pathogen present in the implicated food, usually hours or days after the disease outbreak, during which time there may be significant changes in the size of the inoculum.

Potential for Human Exposure

General Approach. Microorganisms may be transmitted to humans in a variety of ways, including person-to-person transmission, (e.g., through sexual and fecal-oral contact), exposure to air-borne, food-borne, water-borne, and vector-borne pathogens, and contact with contaminated objects. Spread of disease by broiler chickens almost exclusively involves food-borne transmission, although direct contact or air-borne routes may be important in occupational exposures in poultry slaughter and processing plants.

Microorganisms may be introduced into food at a number of points. Many of them, including Campylobacter and Salmonella, are present in the gut flora of animals and may contaminate the surface of the carcass during slaughter or subsequent processing. The actual number of microorganisms present at any one time (and the percentage of carcasses contaminated) may vary widely, depending on temperature, product conditions, and how the product is handled. Most microorganisms are killed during cooking. Infection can occur if the poultry is eaten raw or if parts of it are undercooked. In the kitchen, cooked foods can be contaminated by raw poultry and other foods, by soil, or by food handlers. Once present in a kitchen, these microorganisms may contaminate a variety of foods, including chicken.

Epidemiological studies can often link or attribute outbreaks of food-borne disease to specific products, such as chicken. However, the key point in the chain of transmission generally is the kitchen itself: for most food-borne pathogens, highly contaminated meat will not cause disease if properly cooked and handled. Conversely, minimal contamination can lead to major disease outbreaks if pathogenic microorganisms are allowed to contaminate an entire kitchen and if food prepared in the kitchen is subsequently mishandled.

For many microorganisms, it is possible to measure the level of contamination of a product at each stage of processing. Unfortunately, it is unclear how the level of contamination observed during the processing of such products as raw chicken correlates with the potential for disease transmission. In formal attempts to assess risk, one must recognize the difference between measurable levels of product contamination and disease occurrence. Although the correlation can never be fully resolved, additional data from carefully focused and coordinated epidemiological-microbiological studies could greatly reduce the level of uncertainty.

Sources of Data. The U.S. Department of Agriculture and Food and Drug Administration collect some data on levels of product contamination with certain microorganisms at various stages of processing and distribution. More detailed data, and data on additional microorganisms, have been reported in the literature. Data showing a direct link between product contamination and disease in the community (and subsequent disappearance of disease in association with elimination of contamination) have been published for some microorganisms and some products, but there are few data available on raw chicken or its major pathogens (Bryan, 1980a; CDC, 1983a, b; Horwitz and Gangarosa, 1976).

The CDC collects data on food-borne disease outbreaks through its national food-borne disease surveillance system. As in other national reporting systems and for individual cases of disease, however, there is undoubtedly significant underreporting and an emphasis on more serious illnesses. For example, almost all outbreaks of botulism are reported, whereas outbreaks of other illnesses involving only a few persons with relatively mild symptoms frequently are not investigated or reported. Data on routes of transmission can be obtained from outbreak reports and from case-control studies of specific pathogens. In properly designed case-control studies, it may be possible to determine the percentage of reported cases due to one microorganism that can be attributed to broiler chickens, i.e., attributable risk.

To completely characterize the risk associated with microbial contamination of chicken, there must be sufficient data from which to predict changes in disease occurrence that would result from changes in levels of product contamination at each of several steps from production to the consumer's table. Such data are likely to show an increasing correlation between the potential for diseases to occur and microbial contamination as one moves from production to the ingestion of poultry products. The microbial load on the cooked, ready-to-eat product is the only reliable indicator of disease potential, and the further removed from this point data are obtained, the less reliable they are.

Characterization of Risk

There are sufficient data to clearly establish many microorganisms as a hazard to human health and to estimate (very roughly) the risk of illness associated with eating contaminated chicken. It is also possible to identify where microorganisms may be introduced during processing (see Figures 3-1 and 3-2 in Chapter 3) and to quantitate microbial contamination at those points. These control points, and their identification as part of an HACCP system, have been discussed in detail in a previous report of the National Research Council (NRC, 1985a).

Microorganisms contaminating chicken during processing may die off or reproduce rapidly before reaching the consumer, depending on environmental and product conditions. Thus, levels of contamination on the dinner plate may have little relation to data obtained at the time of slaughter or in the kitchen prior to cooking. Therefore, measurement of the risk posed by microbial contamination of a specific food item, such as chicken, must involve identification and enumeration of cases of illness within an exposure group in addition to sampling during production.

APPLICATION OF METHODS TO INDIVIDUAL AND GROUPS OF POULTRY-BORNE PATHOGENS

Many pathogenic microorganisms have been associated with the production of chickens or with eating chicken. Following are some examples, which are broken down into three general categories:

1. Bacteria known to be pathogenic in humans that are carried on or transmitted by broiler chickens at retail:

Campylobacter jejuni,

Salmonella spp. (excluding S. typhi)

Yersinia enterocolitica

2. Bacteria known to be pathogenic in humans that have been associated with eating chicken:

Bacillus cereus

Clostridium botulinum

Clostridium perfringens

Shigella spp.

Staphylococcus aureus

Contamination by these human pathogens probably occurs during processing and preparation.

3. Microorganisms known to be pathogenic in chickens that are of questionable pathogenic significance for healthy humans when carried on or transmitted by broiler chickens at retail:

Bacteria:

Haemophilus gallinarum

Pasteurella multocida

Escherichia coli

Mycobacterium avium

Mycoplasma spp.

Clostridium colinum

Chlamydia psittaci

Viruses and associated diseases:

Picornavirus (encephalomyelitis)

Alphavirus (equine encephalitis)

Herpesvirus (Marek's disease, infective laryngotracheitis)

Paramyxovirus (Newcastle disease)

Adenovirus (adenoviral tracheitis)

Poxvirus (fowl pox)

Coronavirus (infectious bronchitis)

Orthomyxovirus (avian influenza)

Reovirus (viral arthritis)

Fungi:

Aspergillus spp.

Dactylaria spp.

Parasites:

Cryptosporidium

For some of these microorganisms, their significance as human pathogens and information on their transmission by broiler chickens are discussed in the following paragraphs.

Known Human Pathogens Carried on or Transmitted by Broiler Chickens at Retail

Campylobacter jejuni

Hazard Identification and Evaluation. The gram-negative bacterium Campylobacter jejuni has recently been implicated as one of the most common bacterial causes of gastroenteritis among both children and adults (Pai et al., 1979; Skirrow, 1977). Studies in the United States, Canada, and Europe have demonstrated that C. jejuni is significantly more common in stool samples from patients with diarrhea than in samples from healthy controls (Blaser et al., 1983a). Ingestion of C. jejuni by volunteers has resulted in a clinical diarrheal syndrome (Black et al., 1983; Blaser et al., 1983b).

C. jejuni is pathogenic for normal, healthy adults (Black et al., 1983; Blaser and Reller, 1981). Illness may be more severe in elderly or debilitated patients, and the rare deaths from C. jejuni infection have occurred mostly in that group (Blaser and Reller, 1981). Virulence factors and pathogenic properties of C. jejuni include invasiveness, enterotoxin production, and cytotoxin production (Klipstein et al., 1985). Some investigators have suggested that diarrhea-associated strains are more likely to have one or more of these properties than strains isolated from asymptomatic individuals (Klipstein et al., 1985; Ruiz-Palacios et al., 1983), but these results have not been confirmed by some other investigators (Mathan et al., 1984).

Predominant symptoms among patients identified by positive stool culture include diarrhea, abdominal pain, malaise, fever, nausea, and vomiting (Blaser and Reller, 1981; SKCDPH, 1984). Up to 80% of patients have fever, and approximately 50% give a history of bloody diarrhea (Blaser et al., 1983a; SKCDPH, 1984). Abdominal pain is severe enough to mimic acute appendicitis in about 1% of cases (Skirrow, 1977). Complications rarely include toxic megacolon, gastrointestinal hemorrhage, convulsions (in children with high fevers), a typhoid-like syndrome, meningitis, reactive arthritis (in men with the HLA-B27 histocompatibility antigen), urinary tract infections, and cholecystitis (Blaser and Reller, 1981). Illness is reported most frequently among children less than a year old, and among young adults 20 to 29 years of age (Blaser et al., 1983b; CDSC, 1981; Finch and Riley, 1984; Riley and Finch, 1985).

Illnesses vary widely in severity, ranging from mild diarrhea lasting less than 24 hours to severe bloody diarrhea with abdominal pain and fever lasting several weeks. Some investigators have reported that most patients recover in less than a week (Blaser and Reller, 1981; Butzler and Skirrow, 1979), but a recent study of 225 culture-confirmed cases indicates that the average duration of illness is 13.5 days (SKCDPH, 1984). In that study, 15 (6.7%) of the 225 patients were hospitalized up to 11 days as a result of their infection, most commonly (13 of the 15) for 5 days or less (SKCDPH, 1984).

Since the late 1970s, most clinical microbiology laboratories in the United Kingdom have included cultures for Campylobacter as part of their routine evaluation of stool specimens (CDSC, 1981). In 1981 there were about 12,500 reported isolations of Campylobacter, giving an annual isolation rate of approximately 28 per 100,000 population (Blaser et al., 1983b; CDSC, 1981). Some clinical laboratories in the United States still do not routinely culture stool samples for Campylobacter, and nationwide surveillance for Campylobacter, which began in January 1983, is still not uniformly applied. During the first year, 42 states reported 8,282 isolates of C. jejuni (Riley and Finch, 1985). In all 33 states that participated for at least 11 months in 1983, the number of Campylobacter isolates exceeded the number of Shigella isolates reported. In four states, there were more Campylobacter isolates than Salmonella isolates.

Until national surveillance data are more complete, the best estimates of Campylobacter incidence in the United States will continue to come from laboratories serving defined population groups. In the metropolitan area of Denver, Colorado, investigators found that the annual incidence of reported Campylobacter infections was 17.2 per 100,000 people (Blaser et al., 1983b). In the Seattle-King County Department of Public Health (SKCDPH) study (which did not include active recruitment of patients with diarrhea), the annual incidence was estimated to be 100 per 100,000 (SKCDPH, 1984). For children less than 1 year of age, rates were 332.9 per 100,000 for males and 194.9 per 100,000 for females.

The figures in both of the above studies are based on reported isolation of Campylobacter from stool samples. One study in England projected a 1.1% (1,100 per 100,000) mean annual rate of Campylobacter infection in a defined population (Kendall and Tanner, 1982) or approximately 40 times the reported annual rate of isolations (28 per 100,000). Blaser et al. (1983b) have estimated that in developed countries such as the United States, the incidence of Campylobacter infections, whether symptomatic or not, is about 1% to 2% per year (1,000-2,000 per 100,000). The SKCDPH data (with a relatively high incidence rate) suggest that the annual incidence of hospitalized cases would be approximately 7 per 100,000 if all hospitalized cases in the study population were correctly identified. Data are inadequate to calculate mortality rates (Blaser et al., 1983b).

Dose-Response Studies. For campylobacteriosis, information on dose response is based on a few studies involving small numbers of volunteers and is difficult to interpret. In volunteer studies with C. jejuni strain A3004, for example, 5 of 10 healthy adult volunteers ingesting 8×10^2 colony-forming units (cfu) became infected, and one of the 5 became ill. At 8×10^3 cfu, 6 of 10 were infected, but none were ill. The rate of infection increased with increases in the size of the inoculum until 100% were infected at a dose of 10^8 cfu. At 9×10^4 cfu, the rate of illness was 46%; however, as the size of inoculum was increased, the rate of illness at each dose level ranged from only 9% to 22% (Black et al., 1983). These data, in which the dose varied 100,000-fold, show that risk is far from linear with dose, perhaps because of marked variability in susceptibility.

Epidemiological studies of both person-to-person and water-borne transmission of C. jejuni suggest that relatively small inocula are capable of causing disease (Blaser et al., 1983b). No outbreaks have been reported where it has been possible to clearly associate infection rate with a known inoculum.

Potential for Human Exposure. The prevalence of C. jejuni infection in live broiler chickens is highly variable. Microbiological surveys of live broilers have demonstrated that grow-out premises are inconsistently infected and that infection in one poultry housing unit does not mean that other housing units on the same premises contain infected birds (Smitherman et al., 1984). Within infected flocks, however, infection rates tend to be high, and fecal samples from infected chickens tend to be heavily contaminated (e.g., 10^6 cfu/g of feces) (Grant et al., 1980; Smitherman et al., 1984). C. jejuni has been found at many points during slaughter and processing, and a significant proportion of the broiler chicken carcasses available for retail sale carry the microorganism (Table 4-1).

Persons eating raw or rare chickens contaminated with C. jejuni may ingest sufficient numbers of microorganisms to become infected. Campylobacter can also enter the kitchen via contaminated broiler carcasses and subsequently cross-contaminate other foods. In one study of commercial and institutional kitchens, Hutchinson et al. (1983) found that the hands of workers and kitchen work surfaces often became contaminated with Campylobacter during the preparation of raw chicken. This is similar to the environmental contamination that occurs during the preparation of chicken contaminated by Escherichia coli (De Wit et al., 1979).

Several studies have shown an epidemiological link between chicken and gastroenteritis caused by C. jejuni. Raw chicken eaten by military recruits during a training exercise was implicated in an outbreak in the Netherlands (Brouwer et al., 1979), and ingestion of poorly cooked chicken was associated with illness at a barbecue in Colorado (Blaser et al., 1983b). In another study in Colorado, sporadic illness was associated with the handling of raw chickens in home kitchens (Hopkins and Scott, 1983). Consumption of chicken was associated with sporadic illness in Sweden (Norkrans and Svedham, 1982) and in urban areas of the Federal Republic of Germany (Kist, 1983).

In the SKCDPH (1984) study, significantly more (p = 0.00003) patients with C. jejuni-caused enteritis had eaten chicken than had controls. The relative risk for chicken consumption was 2.4 (95% confidence interval [CI], 1.6-3.6); for rare or raw chicken, it was 7.6 (95% CI, 2.1-27.6); and for cooked chicken, it was 2.3 (95% CI, 1.5-3.5). The method of Walter (1975) was used to estimate that 48.2% of C. jejuni cases were attributable to eating chicken. The link between chicken and human illness was reinforced by finding similarities in antibiograms, plasmid content, and serotypes of C. jejuni isolates taken from poultry at retail and from human cases (SKCDPH, 1984).

Characterization of Risk. The studies cited above indicate that C. jejuni is clearly pathogenic for humans, resulting in as many as 1,000 to 2,000 cases per 100,000 people annually in the United States (Blaser et al., 1983b). Epidemiological studies suggest that at least 48% of Campylobacter cases are attributable to chicken (SKCDPH, 1984).

TABLE 4-1. Rates of Salmonella, Campylobacter, and Yersinia Contamination of Chicken Carcasses

Microorganism	Part of Chicken Sampled and Stage of Procedure	No. Sampled	Percent	Reference
Campylobacter	Chicken livers	40	30	Stern et al., 1984
	Mechanical deboning of chicken	40	12.5	
	Chicken livers from giblet chiller	36	69.4	Wempe et al., 1983
	Wings ready for packaging	36	66.7	
	Wings on arrival at supermarket	94	82.9	Kinde et al., 1983
	Chicken; supermarket shelf	862	23.1	Harris et al., 1986b
Salmonella	Chicken; supermarket shelf	862	4.3	Harris et al., 1986b
	Whole, eviscerated chickens; chill tank exit			Green et al., 1982
	in 1967	597	28.6	
	in 1979	601	36.9	
	Whole, eviscerated chickens; chill tank exit	215	11.6	Campbell et al., 1983
	Whole, eviscerated chickens; chill tank exit	171	20.5	Surkiewicz et al., 1969
Yersinia	Chicken; supermarket shelf	862	1.3	Harris et al., 1986b

Species of Campylobacter are present on a high percentage of chickens at the time of retail sale. Any reduction in the frequency or intensity of contamination may result in a corresponding reduction in the frequency of illness, but the commmittee found no studies that clearly support or refute this hypothesis. Plasmid-mediated resistance to antimicrobial agents has been reported for isolates of C. jejuni isolated from poultry (Bradbury and Munroe, 1985; Harris et al., 1986a, b), and could compromise therapy in infected humans if resistance influences response to a clinically relevant drug.

Nontyphoidal Salmonella Species

Hazard Identification and Evaluation. Salmonella species are among the most common bacterial causes of gastroenteritis in humans. They are found significantly more often in stools of persons with diarrhea than in samples from asymptomatic persons. In studies in volunteers, isolates from the stools of diarrhea patients cause diarrheal disease when fed to humans (McCullough and Eisele, 1951). Normal, healthy adults are susceptible to infection, although illness tends to be more severe among the very young, the very old, or patients with some type of underlying immunosuppression. Certain serotypes or serogroups are characteristically more virulent than others. Putative virulence plasmids have been identified for certain serotypes (Helmuth et al., 1985), but there does not appear to be a single virulence plasmid common to multiple serotypes.

Symptoms usually appear within 6 to 48 hours after ingestion of contaminated food or water. They often begin with nausea and vomiting, followed by diarrhea, abdominal pain, and fever (Blaser et al., 1983a; Hook, 1985; Hornick, 1983). In some cases, the stools may be bloody. Temperature elevations as high as 38° to 39°C are common, as are chills. Abdominal cramps occur in approximately two-thirds of the patients. In severe cases, fluid and electrolyte losses may be profound enough to cause hypovolemic shock. Toxic megacolon has been described as a rare complication (Mandal and Mani, 1976). Transient bacteremia occurs in less than 5% of adults with gastroenteritis, but at a somewhat higher rate in children and persons with major underlying diseases (Hook, 1985; Hyams et al., 1980). Localized suppurative infections (bronchopneumonia, emphysema, endocarditis, pericarditis, arteritis, pyelonephritis, osteomyelitis, arthritis) develop in about 10% of patients with bacteremia (Hook, 1985; Hornick, 1983). Nontyphoidal Salmonella species, particularly S. cholerae-suis, can cause fever and sustained bacteremia without manifestations of enterocolitis (Saphra and Wassermann, 1954).

In the majority of uncomplicated cases, fever lasts for less than 2 days. Diarrhea usually lasts less than 7 days, but occasionally persists for as long as several weeks (Hook, 1985). In the SKCDPH study, mean length of illness was 10.25 days (SKCDPH, 1984). Illness is more severe in children, in the elderly, and in patients who have had a gastrectomy or gastroenterostomy, or who have achlorhydria, sickle-cell anemia, or other conditions that impair resistance to infection.

In food-borne outbreaks, hospitalization rates have ranged from 0 to more than 50%. The CDC (1981) reported that 8% of 2,356 cases in 51 outbreaks reported in 1978 through the CDC Foodborne Disease

Surveillance system were hospitalized. In the SKCDPH (1984) study, 3 (4.1%) of 72 outpatients with positive cultures were later hospitalized.

In Massachusetts, a case-fatality rate of 1.4% was found in a study of 2,600 confirmed cases occurring between 1940 and 1955. A higher mortality rate was seen in older age groups, debilitated patients, and patients with bacteremia (MacCready et al., 1957). A much lower case-fatality rate of 0.1% was observed among 16,172 patients in 261 food-borne outbreaks reported to CDC between 1972 and 1978 (Sours and Smith, 1980).

Salmonellosis has been a reportable disease in the United States since 1942, and data have been collected by CDC through its Salmonella surveillance system since 1963. The incidence of reported cases was approximately 8 per 100,000 in 1963; in 1983, there were approximately 19 cases per 100,000 (CDC, 1984a). Although there are differences by serotype, age-specific rates tend to peak between 2 and 4 months of age at approximately 300 cases per 100,000 and decline rapidly thereafter. After age 5, rates for all serotypes combined remain relatively constant at approximately 10 cases per 100,000 per year (CDC, 1981).

As described for Campylobacter, it is likely that reported cases represent only a small fraction of the total number of infections that occur. From data on outbreaks, it has been estimated that only one in 75 to 100 cases of salmonellosis in the United States is reported (Aserkoff et al., 1970; Hauschild and Bryan, 1980). These types of data indicate that the incidence of actual infections ranges from 1,500 to 2,000 cases per 100,000 population, roughly the same as rates estimated for Campylobacter infections (Blaser et al., 1983b). In the SKCDPH (1984) study, there were 1.4 hospitalized cases of salmonellosis per 100,000 members of the population annually. Similar figures are obtained from reported cases and the percentages of hospitalization reported in studies of outbreaks. The reported number of cases and estimated mortality rates indicate that mortality would range from 0.02 to 0.2 deaths per 100,000 population per year.

Dose-Response Studies. Studies in volunteers have suggested that an inoculum of 10^6 cfu or more is necessary to produce disease (McCullough and Eisele, 1951). However, data from outbreak investigations suggest that the infective dose in nature may be as low as 10^1 to 10^2 cfu (Craven et al., 1975; Silverstolpe et al., 1961). In outbreaks associated with low infective doses, the vehicles of transmission were foods with a high buffering capacity or a high fat content, which may have protected the microorganism from the lethal action of gastric acid (Gangarosa, 1978b).

Potential for Human Exposure. Two relatively host-specific Salmonella serotypes, S. pullorum and S. gallinarum, cause acute or chronic diseases in chickens. S. pullorum, the etiologic agent of pullorum disease in poultry, causes an acute systemic disease that produces a high mortality rate in chicks less than 3 weeks of age, but most often causes a chronic localized disease or may be asymptomatic in older chickens. These two serotypes rarely cause disease in humans.

Infection of chickens by other serotypes of Salmonella most often results in chronic intestinal carriage. These infections occur in poultry worldwide, but the flock incidence is extremely variable (Lee, 1977). Nationwide surveys of market-ready broilers conducted in 1967 and 1979 both demonstrated extreme variability in the contamination rates among various lots of birds, with an incidence range of 7.5% to 73.7% in 1967 and 2.5% to 87.5% in 1979 (Green et al., 1982). Persons eating inadequately cooked chicken infected with Salmonella may ingest sufficient numbers of microorganisms to become infected. The presence of Salmonella on chicken carcasses may also lead to contamination of the kitchen environment and other foods.

Characterization of Risk. Salmonella clearly causes disease in humans. Projections from available data suggest that there are between 1,500 to 2,000 cases per 100,000 members of the population per year. Data on attributable risk are not as complete as those for C. jejuni, but numerous epidemiological studies document a major role for broiler chickens as a vehicle for salmonellosis in humans. Salmonella is present on chickens, and many studies have documented the points at which contamination occurs during production and processing. At the time of retail sale, a high percentage of chickens bear Salmonella (CDC, 1977, 1983b, 1984b, 1985). A reduction in the frequency or degree of contamination of chicken with Salmonella would logically result in a reduction in human disease; however, as for C. jejuni, there are no quantitative data linking contamination levels with disease occurrence. Thus, it is not known with certainty whether a reduction in Salmonella on broiler chickens would have any appreciable influence on the incidence of salmonellosis. In the absence of such data, it is not possible to do a quantitative assessment of the public health risk posed by specific levels of Salmonella on chicken carcasses.

Yersinia enterocolitica

Hazard Identification and Evaluation. Yersinia enterocolitica is recognized as a significant cause of acute enteritis and enterocolitis (Bottone, 1977). It may also cause mesenteric adenitis, hepatosplenic abscesses, or septicemia, and may initiate a variety of autoimmune processes, including erythema nodosum and polyarthritis (Anonymous, 1984; Bottone, 1977). There is some evidence implicating Y. enterocolitica in Reiter's syndrome, carditis, glomerulonephritis, Grave's disease, and Hashimoto's thyroiditis (Anonymous, 1984; Larsen, 1980). Host factors appear to play a major role in pathogenicity and in the expression of yersiniosis: diarrhea is seen more frequently in young children, mesenteric adenitis in older children and adolescents, and autoimmune phenomena in women. Arthritis correlates with occurrence of the HLA B27 histocompatibility antigen.

Illness has been associated with the isolation of Y. enterocolitica from clinical specimens in several outbreak investigations (Black et al., 1978; Shayegani et al., 1983; Tacket et al., 1985). At least one case-control study showed an association between the occurrence of diarrhea and isolation of the microorganism (Marks et al., 1980). Chronic Yersinia infection can be established by history and serologic evidence of prior infection (Anonymous, 1984). There are no good data on Y. enterocolitica infections from studies in volunteers. Given the invasive nature of the microorganism and the potential seriousness of infections, it is unlikely that such data could be obtained at this time.

The pathogenicity of Y. enterocolitica appears to depend on several factors, including the presence of the O serogroup and invasive strains of plasmids ranging in molecular mass from 40 to 48 megadaltons (Gemski et al., 1980; Portnoy et al., 1981). Disease-associated Y. enterocolitica strains isolated in Europe have generally belonged to serogroups 0:3 and 0:9 (de Groote et al., 1982). In the United States serogroup 0:8 is the most common serogroup isolated, but this pattern may be changing (Bottone, 1983). The invasive strains of plasmids encode, among other properties, the production of specific outer membrane proteins, calcium dependence, and adherence to HEp-2 tissue culture cells (Heesemann et al., 1984); other proposed virulence factors, including invasion of HeLa cells and enterotoxin production, appear to be chromosomally mediated (Kay et al., 1983; Schiemann and Devenish, 1982). At this time no single factor appears to be sufficient to differentiate pathogenic from nonpathogenic strains (Kay et al., 1983).

Laboratories in the United States that routinely culture all stool samples report isolation rates for Y. enterocolitica in stools, blood, and other samples that are only about 3.8% to 33.6% of the rate for Salmonella (Marymont et al., 1982; Snyder et al., 1982). Studies in Europe suggest that stool isolates account for more than 95% of total Yersinia isolates. Extrapolating from the previously cited data on Salmonella (approximately 19 reported cases per 100,000 per year), and assuming that there are 5% as many Yersinia isolates as Salmonella isolates, the incidence of diagnosed Yersinia infections would be approximately one per 100,000 members of the population per year. In the absence of good data relating total infection rates to diagnosed infections, it is not possible to predict the actual number of infections that may occur. Up to 30% of isolates of Y. enterocolitica are obtained from hospitalized patients, and as much as 10% of reported infections may be associated with a syndrome of mesenteric adenitis mimicking appendicitis (de Groote et al., 1982; Snyder et al., 1982; Tacket et al., 1985). These data suggest that hospitalization rates are proportionately much higher than those resulting from Salmonella infections (1-2%). Data are inadequate to calculate mortality rates accurately.

Dose-Response Studies. Because of the potential seriousness of yersiniosis, studies of infectious doses have not been performed on large numbers of volunteers. Enterocolitis and fever resulted in one person who ingested 3.5×10^9 organisms. The symptoms lasted for 4 weeks (Szita et al., 1973). In epidemiological studies, the necessity of using the standard microbiological enrichment procedures for contaminated specimens makes it difficult to estimate levels of contamination from epidemiologically linked foods.

Potential for Human Exposure. Investigators who have specifically looked for colonization of Y. enterocolitica have identified the microorganism in a small percentage of broiler chickens available for retail sale. Y. enterocolitica has also been isolated from a variety of sources, including wild and domestic animals and water (Vantrappen et al., 1982) as well as poultry, beef, pork, fish, oysters, raw milk, and pasteurized milk (Lee, 1977; Morris and Feeley, 1976; Rechtman et al., 1985; Schiemann and Toma, 1978; Stengel, 1985).

Characterization of Risk. The widespread presence of Yersinia in the environment and the diversity of food vehicles potentially involved in food-borne outbreaks suggest that broiler chickens may not be a major source of yersiniosis in humans, despite the microorganism's presence on chickens in retail stores. Better data are needed on the roles of various foodstuffs, including poultry, in the epidemiology of yersiniosis.

Known Human Pathogens Associated with the Ingestion of Chicken

Campylobacter, Salmonella, and Yersinia are not the only pathogens associated with eating chicken. Generally, however, raw chicken does not appear to be a major channel through which other pathogenic microorganisms enter the kitchen. Spore-forming microorganisms such as Bacillus cereus, Clostridium botulinum, and C. perfringens appear to be ubiquitous in nature. Although they may be present on the surface of chickens, they are as likely, or more likely, to be brought into the kitchen in soil or on vegetables, grains, or other farm products. Shigella , which is infectious at very low doses, tends to be transmitted by direct fecal-oral contact. For example, it may be transferred directly onto food by food handlers whose hands have been contaminated with feces containing the microorganism. Isolates of Shigella boydii have infrequently been obtained from poultry feces (Fagerberg and Quarles, 1982). The direct role of consumer-ready chicken in human shigellosis is unclear, but is probably negligible. Staphylococci tend to be transferred to food by persons whose hands are infected with staphylococci or by people who are chronic nasal or rectal carriers of the microorganism. Two species in this group, B. cereus and C. botulinum, are described in detail in the following paragraphs. A full formal risk assessment will require similar analyses of other pathogens in this category.

Bacillus Cereus

Hazard Identification and Evaluation. Bacillus cereus is an aerobic, spore-forming, gram-positive rod that has recently been implicated as a cause of gastroenteritis. High counts of B. cereus have been detected in food implicated in disease outbreaks and, less often, in stool samples from ill patients. There are no data showing an association between B. cereus and cases of sporadic diarrhea, although up to 14% of asymptomatic persons in the general population may have the microorganism in their stool (Ghosh, 1978). There have been limited volunteer experiments with this microorganism. Hauge (1955) inoculated vanilla sauce with a strain of B. cereus isolated from an outbreak of food poisoning in Norway, and ingested about 200 ml of the sauce containing approximately 10^{10} microorganisms; 13 hours later he experienced severe abdominal pain, diarrhea, and rectal tenesmus, which persisted for 8 hours. In a previous experiment, four of six other volunteers who drank 155 to 270 ml of vanilla sauce containing 30 to 60 million B. cereus per milliliter experienced similar symptoms (Gilbert, 1979; Hauge, 1950).

Two clinical syndromes are associated with B. cereus: a short incubation vomiting syndrome (similar to that seen with staphylococcal food poisoning) associated with a heat-stable emetic toxin and a diarrheal syndrome (similar to that seen with Clostridium perfringens) associated with production of a heat-labile, cyclic AMP-mediated enterotoxin (Terranova and Blake, 1978). B. cereus has also been implicated as a cause of bacteremia, pneumonia, and meningitis, and has been isolated from serious wound infections in otherwise healthy patients as well as from immunocompromised patients (Turnbull et al., 1977, 1979).

B. cereus has been widely recognized in Europe as an important cause of food-borne disease. Between 1960 and 1966, for example, B. cereus was the third most commonly reported cause of food-borne disease outbreaks in Hungary (Goepfert et al., 1972). Such outbreaks have been identified infrequently in the United States, however. Of approximately 1,800 food-borne disease outbreaks of known etiology reported to CDC between 1966 and 1979, only 19 were attributed to B. cereus, including 10 outbreaks of the diarrheal syndrome and 9 of the emetic syndrome (Morris, 1981). These numbers probably reflect severe underrecognition of B. cereus outbreaks. Most laboratories in the United States are not familiar with the microorganism and do not attempt to isolate it routinely from stool and food samples.

Dose-Response Studies. There are inadequate data to clearly establish an infectious dose for B. cereus. Doses of 10^{10} have caused disease in rhesus monkeys and volunteers. Counts higher than 105 per gram of food have been associated with disease in outbreak investigations (Morris, 1981).

Potential for Human Exposure. B. cereus is ubiquitous in soil and can be isolated from virtually all farm produce, including vegetables

(51.2% of samples in one study [Nygren, 1962]), grain (91.2% of uncooked rice samples [Gilbert and Parry, 1977]), and milk and dairy products (including, in one study, 86.7% of bottled pasteurized milk samples [Gilbert, 1979; Ionescu et al., 1966]). It is also common in dried and processed foods, including spices (72.3% of samples [Nygren, 1962]) and products such as chocolate pudding powder (46% of samples tested [Nygren, 1962]) and dried chicken (47.8% of samples [Nygren, 1962]). Outbreaks of the vomiting syndrome have almost all been associated with fried rice; conditions inside rice warmers used in Chinese restaurants appear to be ideal for germination, growth, and production of the emetic toxin (Gilbert et al., 1974).

Chicken has been implicated as the vehicle of B. cereus transmission in at least one outbreak of diarrheal disease in the United States (Midura et al., 1970) and in several other outbreaks reported in the literature, but there are no good data on rates of isolation from raw chicken (Gilbert, 1979). Data are not adequate to determine whether contamination of chickens before or after retail sale played a role in these outbreaks, and there are no data to suggest that chickens play a more significant role than other foods in the transmission of B. cereus.

Characterization of Risk. The wide distribution of B. cereus in the environment and in various foods suggests that contaminated broiler chickens are not a major factor in the spread of this microorganism. An accurate assessment of the public health risk attributable to broiler chickens would require additional knowledge of the epidemiological characteristics of disease caused by food-borne B. cereus.

Clostridium botulinum

Hazard Identification and Evaluation. Investigators have demonstrated a clear association between the presence of botulinal toxin in food and human illness. Group I, II, and possibly IV (types A, B, E, F, and G) toxins produced by Clostridium botulinum are responsible for the neurologic signs and symptoms observed in human cases of botulism (Morris and Hatheway, 1983). No well-documented studies of food-borne botulism in volunteers have been conducted. When botulinal toxin is used to treat strabismus in humans, however, it is known to cause localized paralysis after injection into muscle (Scott, 1981).

Botulism patients typically have blurred vision as well as difficulty speaking and swallowing. During the 24 to 72 hours after onset, there may also be a progressive descending motor paralysis, resulting, in the most severe cases, in total loss of motor function, including respiratory function (Hughes et al., 1981; Morris and Hatheway, 1983). Recovery is usually complete in patients who receive adequate supportive care, including mechanical respiratory support. The average duration of respiratory support is 1 month, but has been provided for as long as 7 months (Morris and Hatheway, 1983).

Between 1950 and 1979, approximately 25 cases of food-borne botulism were reported in the United States each year (CDC, 1979). Virtually all these patients were hospitalized. The case-fatality rate for botulism is currently less than 10%, down from approximately 70% between 1910 and 1919. This improvement is attributable primarily to the widespread availability of long-term respiratory support (Morris and Hatheway, 1983).

Dose-Response Studies. In contrast to most other food-borne diseases, botulism is caused by the presence of toxin in food, rather than by the ingestion of the microorganisms themselves. Consequently, disease severity is directly related to the amount of toxin present in the food. A dose of 10^{-8} g of purified botulinal toxin is probably sufficient to cause disease in a human; doses between 10^{-6} and 10^{-7} g can be a lethal (Morris and Hatheway, 1983).

Potential for Human Exposure. C. botulinum spores are widely distributed in the environment and may be isolated from soils and marine sediments, the surfaces of vegetables and fruit, and fish and other seafood. To germinate, spores require anaerobic conditions (restricted oxygen and sufficiently low Eh [redox potential]), adequate nutrients, low acidity (pH > 4.6), sufficient availability of water (low solute concentrations; Aw [water activity] 0.93), suitable temperature, and lack of inhibiting substances. If spores are present on food maintained under such conditions (e.g., in improperly home-canned food), they will germinate and toxin will be released as vegetative cells lyse. The toxin is heat labile and is destroyed by cooking (Morris and Hatheway, 1983).

Chicken or chicken-containing products were implicated as the vehicle of infection in 4 of the 190 outbreaks of food-borne botulism of known etiology reported between 1950 and 1977 (CDC, 1979). These included two outbreaks resulting from the consumption of commercially prepared chicken pot pie (one from type A toxin and one from a toxin of an undetermined type), one outbreak involving commercially prepared chicken livers (type A toxin), and one involving home-canned chicken soup (type B toxin). Given the heat-lability of the toxin, mishandling of the product (and subsequent toxin production) most likely occurred after initial cooking. Although chicken carcasses may occasionally carry C. botulinum spores, there are no data to suggest that this has any significant effect on the occurrence of disease in the human population.

Chickens are themselves susceptible to botulism. Type C toxin (produced by group III C. botulinum growing in decaying vegetation or decomposing carcasses) causes limberneck (a disease characterized by diffuse motor paralysis) in chickens, turkeys, and several species of wild birds. Apparently, type C toxin can also affect mammals, and there are at least two poorly documented reports of type C disease in humans (Hariharan and Mitchell, 1977). There are no data to suggest that humans have acquired type C disease by eating affected birds; even if affected birds were eaten, cooking should destroy any toxin present in the tissue.

Characterization of Risk. The risk to humans presented by preformed botulinal toxin in raw chicken appears to be negligible. Botulinal spores may be carried on raw chicken, but given the wide distribution of spores in the environment, there is no evidence that this is associated with an increased risk of illness.

Microorganisms Known to be Pathogenic in Chickens That Are of Questionable Significance as Food-Borne Pathogens Transmitted by Broiler Chickens

Many other microorganisms, including bacteria, viruses, and parasites, are common causes of disease in poultry but play an uncertain role in human disease. Host-specificity appears to preclude many of these microorganisms from contributing to the burden of food-borne disease in humans. Other microorganisms, such as Chlamydia psittaci, may cause disease in humans, but are transmitted through routes other than oral. Still others, such as Mycobacterium avium, are shared by humans and poultry, but there is no evidence that broiler chickens serve as a vehicle for transmitting this microorganism to humans.

This section provides examples of the information necessary to assess the risk to public health posed by the microorganisms in this group. Inasmuch as new human enteric pathogens continue to be identified, a more thorough and continuing review of avian pathogens should be a part of a complete public health risk assessment of broiler chicken inspection.

Bacteria. Haemophilus gallinarum causes infectious coryza in poultry, and some strains kill mice when injected intraperitoneally, but it does not appear to be pathogenic in humans (McGaughey, 1932). Infectious coryza is relatively common among the diseases of broilers, but the affinity of the agent for upper airway tissues, which are removed during slaughter and processing, should keep contamination low even in severely affected birds.

Pasteurella multocida causes fowl cholera in domestic poultry. Most avian strains belong to capsular type A, but some are type D; both of these antigenic types can cause respiratory disease in humans (Carter, 1962, 1972; Smith, 1955). Although outbreaks of fowl cholera can occur in flocks, P. multocida is transmitted to humans mainly by inhalation of infectious aerosols emanating from coughing poultry or livestock. Thus, it presents an occupational risk of respiratory disease rather than a risk of food-borne infection to the consumer.

Infection of broilers by Escherichia coli is an important cause of several clinical syndromes. E. coli is also an important cause of disease in humans, different serotypes typically being identified with different pathogenic mechanisms (Gangarosa, 1978a; Gangarosa and Merson, 1977; Guerrant, 1980). There is some overlap between 0 group serotypes isolated from diseased poultry and those characterized as enteropathogenic, enterotoxigenic, and enteroinvasive for humans, but data are inadequate to determine whether E. coli strains from poultry are important contributors to food-borne disease (Glantz, 1971; Gross, 1983). Better definitions of the extent to which E. coli causes enteric disease in humans and the role of contaminated poultry as a vehicle are needed.

Clostridium colinum is associated with ulcerative enteritis in young chickens. This is not particularly common in the broiler industry, and no evidence was found to suggest a pathogenic role for C. colinum in humans (Borriella, 1985).

Species of Mycoplasma are found mainly in the oral cavity, the upper respiratory tract, and distal genital tract of humans and birds, and are host-specific (Hayflick, 1969). Therefore, although M. gallisepticum is a major contributor to chonic respiratory disease in chickens and M. synoviae causes both respiratory disease and infectious synovitis in poultry, current knowledge does not suggest that they pose a health hazard to consumers of broiler chickens.

Nontuberculous mycobacteria, including those in the Mycobacterium avium complex, cause chronic pulmonary disease, lymphadenitis, other soft tissue infections, and bone and joint disease in humans (Wolinsky, 1979). Immunosuppressed individuals and those with underlying chronic lung disease are especially susceptible (Damsker and Bottone, 1985; Good, 1985). Infection in poultry is caused by serotypes 1, 2, and 3 (Thoen et al., 1981), but clinically evident disease is restricted almost entirely to old laying hens. Therefore, in countries where extensive long-term hen holding is not practiced, e.g., in the United States, human infections with M. avium complex microorganisms are due primarily to strains other than the avian serotypes 1, 2, and 3 (Meissner and Anz, 1977; Schaefer, 1968). For this group of microorganisms, the sources and vehicles of human infections need further investigation In many cases, they appear to be of environmental origin (e.g., from water, sand, and sawdust) (Meissner and Anz, 1977; Schaefer, 1968).

In humans, Chlamydia psittaci can cause infections ranging from asymptomatic to severe systemic disease. Most uncompromised people who become ill have only a flu-like syndrome, but infections in the elderly can be life-threatening (Kuritsky et al., 1984). Of the 100 to 150 cases of psittacosis in humans reported in the United States each year, most are associated with caged pet birds (Potter and Kaufmann, 1979). Headache, chills, and fever are the most commonly reported symptoms. Roentgenographic evidence of pneumonitis is found commonly in patients with little clinical evidence of pulmonary lesions (Kuritsky et al., 1984). Chickens are susceptible to infection by C. psittaci , but such infections are rare. Nearly all poultry-associated cases of psittacosis in humans appear to result from occupational exposure to infected turkeys during slaughtering (Anderson et al., 1978; Durfee et al., 1975; Filstein et al., 1981; Hines et al., 1957; Meyer and Eddie, 1942). There is no evidence that market-ready chickens present a risk for psittacosis in humans.

Avian Viruses. There are numerous reports on infection of humans by the paramyxovirus that causes Newcastle disease in poultry. One hundred cases of Newcastle disease virus (NDV) infections in humans were reported from 1943 to 1958 (Chang, 1981), but there have been fewer reports in the more recent medical literature. Of the three types of NDV, two (lentogenic and velogenic viruses) have been reported to cause infection in humans (Dardiri et al., 1962; Miller and Yates, 1971; Reagan et al., 1956). The most common symptom of these infections is a unilateral conjunctivitis, which lasts for 3 to 4 days. Bilateral conjunctivitis, chills, malaise, headache, and fever have also been reported. Newcastle disease in humans is considered to be an occupational hazard for those who have close contact with poultry and for laboratory personnel who work with the virus. There is no evidence that ingestion of meat contaminated with NDV causes infection of humans.

Strains of influenza A viruses infect humans and a large variety of birds, including chickens (Murphy and Webster, 1985; Wood et al., 1985). The common antigenic components of these strains (e.g., Asian H2N2) suggest that avian species may have been involved in the origin of the Asian virus that affects humans (Kaplan, 1980; Nerome et al., 1984). The avian influenza outbreak in chickens that occurred in Pennsylvania and surrounding states from October 1983 through February 1984 was associated with H5N2 influenza A viruses. People in direct contact with infected birds were shown to carry the avian virus over a short period, but there was no evidence that they developed infections (Bean et al., 1985).

The avian retroviruses, such as avian leukosis virus (ALV), cause a variety of neoplastic diseases in chickens (Crittenden, 1976; Fenner et al., 1974). The chick embryos used in the production of yellow fever vaccine during World War II were contaminated with ALV, but thus far, no association has been found between immunization with vaccines containing oncogenic ALV and leukemia, lymphoma, or other cancers in humans (Richman et al., 1972; Waters et al., 1972). Researchers have found no etiologic relationship between avian and human leukemia (Solomon and Purchase, 1969), no evidence of ALV group-specific antibodies in human serum (Roth and Dougherty, 1971), and no association between cancers in humans and avian myeloblastosis virus (Hehlmann et al., 1972). There is also no evidence that ALV and related viruses are infectious or carcinogenic in humans.

Arboviral encephalitides in mammals (including humans) and birds are caused by alphaviruses. These viruses are transmitted by a mosquito vector. Thus, although both chickens and humans are susceptible to infection by both Eastern and Western equine encephalitis viruses, meat from infected broiler chickens would not present a food-borne hazard to consumers.

The medical literature provides no evidence that Marek's disease herpesvirus (MDV) is pathogenic for humans. Relatively high titers of anti-MDV antibody were found in 64 samples of human sera by Naito et al. (1970). In a similar study, however, investigators found no significant anti-MDV antibody titers in 205 serum samples from persons who worked with the virus in laboratories or who had contact with infected chickens (Sharma et al., 1973). Other serologic studies to obtain evidence of MDV infections in humans have produced negative results, both in healthy individuals and in cancer patients (Makari, 1973; Purchase and Witter, 1986).

The committee found no evidence of human infection by avian reoviruses, poxviruses, adenoviruses, or avian infectious bronchitis virus. Although avian infectious laryngotracheitis virus is not known to infect humans, a related herpesvirus has been reported to cause subacute myelo-opticoneuropathy in humans in Japan (Biggs, 1982; Inoue, 1973, 1975; Inoue and Nishibe, 1973; Nishimura and Tobe, 1973; Roizman and Batterson, 1985).

Parasites. Since its recognition as a human pathogen in 1976, Cryptosporidium has been identified as an important cause of diarrheal disease worldwide (Navin, 1985). In humans, cryptosporidiosis is generally manifested as a short-term cholera-like diarrheal illness in immunocompetent people or as a prolonged life-threatening illness in immunodeficient patients (Current, 1985). Among immunocompetent people, the infection appears to be more common in children than in adults. In poultry, Cryptosporidium has been associated with mild intestinal disease and severe respiratory tract disease. Although early studies documented the potential for bird-to-human transmission (Current, 1985), most Cryptosporidium infections in humans are probably not acquired directly from infected birds (Navin, 1985). The frequency with which these cases are due to person-to-person, water-borne, or food-borne transmission is unknown.

USING THE RISK MODEL TO DEVELOP PROGRAMS AND STRATEGIES

The need to reduce the public health risk associated with microbial contamination of foods, including poultry products, has been clearly established. Reports to the CDC during the past 10 years indicated that outbreaks of illnesses attributable to the ingestion of chicken have included infections and intoxications due to Salmonella spp., Campylobacter jejuni, Shigella spp., Staphylococcus aureus, Clostridium perfringens, Bacillus cereus, and Clostridium botulinum. Archer and Kvenberg (1985) estimated that millions of cases of food-borne illnesses costing billions of dollars occur each year. It has also been well documented that various known and potential pathogens can contaminate the poultry product at different stages of production, from transovarial infection of eggs by Salmonella (Faddoul and Fellows, 1966) to contamination of carcasses or parts by environmental Clostridium perfringens during further processing or preparation for consumption (Bryan, 1980b). Managing the risks produced in such divergent ways by microorganisms with such diverse characteristics requires careful application of the precepts of formal risk assessment and risk management.

Analysis of the data with the tools of risk assessment would permit FSIS to validate the assumptions made during the preceding risk assessment, to determine the relative effectiveness of alternative risk management tools, and to establish priorities for each activity in the subsequent program period. Regular reevaluation of priorities would permit FSIS to take advantage of emerging technologies to manage new public health risks. Through continual reassessment, it would be possible to identify and replace inspection methods that had outlived their usefulness without disrupting program continuity.

As discussed in Chapter 3, before a rational program to manage the risk of poultry-borne disease can be developed, one must first have data derived from a comprehensive risk assessment. The activities necessary for the collection of such data are discussed below along with proposed risk-management options.

Risk Assessment

Activity 1. Identification of Potential Pathogens on Broiler Chickens . Bacteria, fungi, protozoa, and viruses may be associated with chickens, either producing disease or living as commensals. These microorganisms can infect poultry during production or can become contaminants during slaughter, processing, and further handling. Microorganisms present in or on chickens have been described by several groups (NRC, 1969, 1985b) and in the first section of this report. To supplement this information, it would be desirable to collect and analyze end product contamination data, i.e., what microorganisms does the consumer encounter at the time broiler chickens are purchased or consumed?

Such data can be obtained in part from reviews of the scientific literature. For example, Todd (1980) reviewed the world literature published during the 1960s and 1970s and found extremely variable rates of contamination of fresh and frozen chicken by Salmonella. This author also described other microbial contaminants of market-ready poultry. Numerous reports of infectious diseases of poultry appear annually in journals of veterinary medicine and poultry science. Each year, for example, Avian Diseases, the journal of the American Association of Avian Pathologists, contains diagnostic summaries from selected laboratories that diagnose poultry disease. From 1981 to 1983, these summaries included more than 30 infectious diseases and conditions that should be considered in a complete risk assessment. Journals covering food science and microbiology also contain reports on microbial contaminants of poultry and edible poultry products.

A second and equally important source of data is the careful analysis of FSIS microbiological surveys. The data should be supplemented by the collection of additional specific critical data, such as determination of the level of microbial contamination in condemned birds—something recommended in a previous NRC report (NRC, 1985a). These comparative data on microbial contamination of passed and condemned carcasses are needed for evaluation of inspection procedures.

Data can also be obtained from field studies of stores and homes. Although FSIS authority beyond processing is limited, field studies are critical to its major mission, i.e., to ensure the sound and effective use of inspection to protect the public health. These studies should include a quantitative component so that microorganisms present only intermittently on a small percentage of chickens (or present only at very low levels) can be distinguished from microorganisms found persistently on a high percentage of carcasses, and contamination levels can be compared over time, between and within geographic areas, from flock to flock, and in other ways related either to human disease or to possible control measures.

These data will permit the development of a comprehensive list of microorganisms present on broiler chickens and will indicate what further risk-assessment data are needed. Quantitative data are necessary in the risk-assessment process itself.

This information should be continually updated as new reports are published and results are obtained from a well-designed FSIS surveillence system. Careful review of the data should lead to the identification of critical gaps in the data base and to the initiation of new studies to provide the needed information. Data from the rapidly maturing field of avian microbiology should be continually integrated into FSIS risk-assessment processes.

Activity 2: Collection of Data Necessary for Risk Assessment. Formal risk assessments should be conducted for each potentially hazardous microorganism by using the format outlined in this chapter. The resulting data should be as accurate and comprehensive as possible to support a formal determination about the risk-management strategy that should be applied. The data may indicate that some microorganisms do not require risk management if they are judged to present minimal risk, if they are not pathogenic in humans, or if their presence in broiler chickens is not important in the epidemiology of human diseases. Other microorganisms (e.g., Salmonella and Campylobacter) may be judged to be important public health risks, because data support an important role for poultry as a vehicle of food-borne disease in consumers. These microorganisms will be considered in the further development of risk-management strategies.

For many microorganisms known to be pathogenic in chickens, there are only limited data on the risk to human health. For microorganisms that are known human pathogens, such as Yersinia spp., more careful assessment of the potential for human exposure is needed; for example, evaluation of data on product contamination levels and acquisition of data on attributable risk (i.e., what percentage of cases can be attributed to chickens) similar to the study of Campylobacter conducted by the Seattle-King County Department of Public Health for FDA (SKCDPH, 1984).

By using the data developed in this activity, one should be able to identify and establish priorities for managing high-risk microorganisms that are on or in broiler chickens at retail, are known to be human pathogens, and are transmitted through food. These priorities should guide FSIS in its management of microbial risks to public health. In particular, they should carry implications regarding the kinds and intensities of inspection that would be most appropriate. For example, what portion of available resources should be devoted to microbiological inspection? How much does organoleptic inspection reduce microbial risks? Would a sampling program, combined with an FSIS and industry shift from detection to prevention, provide enhanced protection? These and related questions will require the best possible quantitative risk assessments. Thus, the priority list will have substantial importance. From the data reviewed in this chapter, it is likely that the list would include Salmonella, Campylobacter, and possibly Yersinia.

Activity 3: Determination of Major Control Points. As a first step toward risk management, efforts should be made to determine the major control points for each high-risk microorganism by using the flow diagrams given in Chapter 3. In general, the control points can be grouped into two major categories: those that influence the level of microbial contamination at the time of retail sale and those that dictate levels at the time the product is consumed (the so-called dinner plate count). It would clearly be advantageous if microbial contamination could be totally eliminated before retail sale or before consumption, but complete control at either stage is unlikely. For example, total elimination of microorganisms such as Salmonella from chicken carcasses does not appear to be likely at present, nor is it likely that mishandling of chickens by consumers can ever be completely prevented.

If complete control cannot be achieved, the problem then becomes one of assessing the relative importance of each of these areas (or each group of control points) as determinants of disease. While studies have demonstrated a great deal of fluctuation in the levels of microbial contamination during processing, contamination at the time of sale can be directly measured and should be susceptible to modification by using an HACCP system explicitly designed for the control of each microorganism within the framework of production practices in each slaughter facility.

The HACCP systems would undoubtedly have some effect on disease incidence, but the limited studies reviewed in this chapter do not show a clear relationship between reduced contamination levels and the occurrence of illness. Numerous studies have documented both the expense and the frustration of trying to control microbial contamination of poultry and suggest that very strict guidelines for limiting microbial contamination during processing may not provide commensurate health benefits.

There is a need for additional quantitative data relating disease incidence to microbial contamination at the time of retail sale. Unfortunately, however, the development of such data is not easy. One approach, which has already been applied, is based on the use of a large health maintenance organization in conjunction with a population-based surveillance system (SKCDPH, 1984). An alternative approach, which offers the advantage of providing a broader-based population sample and a quantifiable risk, would be based on a system of sentinel county health departments in counties where broiler chickens are supplied almost entirely from a few identified processing plants. The county would require a public health infrastructure that includes centralized laboratory facilities and prompt reporting to the epidemiologist in charge; microbiological competence for isolating and identifying specified pathogens; and the ability to perform epidemiological studies adequately so that risk factors can be identified for each infection found. Data on disease incidence in these counties could then be correlated with FSIS microbiological survey data, thereby permitting direct correlation of illness rates and microbial contamination levels. These sentinel counties could also be used to test the relative impact of changes in inspection strategies and the efficacy of control programs for specific microorganisms.

Risk Management

As outlined in the 1985 NRC report on meat and poultry inspection (NRC, 1985b), programs to limit microbial contamination during processing of broiler chickens are best considered as part of an HACCP system. The success of such programs can be measured directly by end-product sampling; however, there is also a need for data of the type described above if changes in microbial contamination are to be related to the occurrence of disease in the community (i.e., to public health).

There has been considerable debate concerning the advisability and feasibility of classifying raw foods of animal origin as either acceptable or unacceptable on the basis of microbiological criteria. To justify the establishment of regulatory standards, such as mandatory limits on the frequency or numbers of specified pathogenic microorganisms, statistically defensible background data and a clearly defined need are necessary. There are clear deficiencies in the data base on poultry-borne disease in the United States. Therefore, this committee concurs with the earlier NRC committee (NRC, 1985a) that microbiological standards for pathogens in raw poultry are inappropriate at this time. The committee does, however, encourage FSIS and the industry to begin exploring strategies to decrease the levels of fecal contamination of edible poultry tissue to improve the overall microbial quality while new data are being generated.

The production of Salmonella-free poultry could serve as the first line of defense against salmonellosis (Linton, 1983). Programs to eradicate S. gallinarum and S. pullorum in poultry have been largely successful, but attempts to eliminate other serotypes in poultry have been less so, largely because of the multiplicity of sources, the complexity of transmission, and the lack of coordination among groups responsible for control at different points.

Control of microorganisms that are not host-adapted will be similar for <u>Salmonella</u> serotypes and other microorganisms. In defining critical control points, consideration should be given to a number of factors, including facility design; isolation of broilers; controlled access to poultry houses, feed, water, litter, breeding stock, and eggs; cleaning and disinfection; and availability of veterinary diagnosis for sick or dead birds. Careful control of these points has been shown to effect large reductions in the prevalence of salmonellosis in turkeys (Campbell et al., 1982).

In slaughter and processing facilities, clean equipment and good sanitation are essential to prevent contamination of edible poultry tissues by intestinal flora and environmental microorganisms. Many investigators have attempted to measure the levels of contaminants on poultry carcasses at various points in the slaughter or processing chain, most often for <u>Salmonella,</u> and have shown that microbial loads are established early in the slaughter process (Campbell et al., 1984). Carcasses are chilled in a common cold water bath, but if the chillers are operated properly, there is little opportunity for cross-contamination, as demonstrated by the Commission of European Communities (CEC, 1976), which reported that reduction of contamination before chilling was more important than the type of chilling procedures used. Other possible sources of contamination and cross-contamination of carcasses during slaughter and processing should be similarly studied to determine where and when contamination is introduced or exacerbated so that the principles of the HACCP system can be applied to reduce the microbial load on the market-ready broiler.

Consumer handling of broiler chickens after retail purchase plays a major role in determining whether microorganisms present at the time of purchase will cause human disease. The principles of good food handling are relatively simple: chicken should always be thoroughly cooked, efforts should be made to minimize cross-contamination within the kitchen, and food should be kept either warm, at least to 140°F (60°C), or cold, below 40°F (4.44°c), to minimize multiplication of potential food-borne pathogens.

A range of programs could be developed, or current programs expanded, to educate consumers about the importance of good food-handling practices. This might include increased emphasis on school education programs, development of adult consumer education materials, dessemination of information on public or commercial television or radio, or the development of product inserts describing proper handling techniques for poultry. Given the frequency of food-borne disease outbreaks associated with restaurants and institutions, efforts should also be directed toward reenforcing the importance of correct food-handling practices in those establishments.

It is much more difficult to assess the final outcome of educational programs than to assess programs to limit microbial contamination during processing. However, it would be possible to pretest the public health impact of major programs in all these areas by using a community-based surveillance system, as described above. The proposed educational programs for food handlers or homemakers could be instituted in such counties, and their subsequent impact on disease incidence could be measured directly.

IMPLICATIONS OF THE PROPOSED RISK MODEL FOR MICROBIAL CONTAMINATION FOR THE CURRENT FSIS INSPECTION PROGRAM

The committee believes that the present system of inspection does very little to protect the public against microbial hazards in broiler chickens. The issue of whether bird-by-bird inspection offers greater public health protection than would inspection of a sample has not been addressed in a rigorous scientific manner. Likewise, microbiological differences between passed and condemned carcasses have not been demonstrated. Furthermore, the public health impact of current inspection procedures has not been defined. In the absence of such data, the committee recommends that FSIS begin now to lay the groundwork for a shift of resources from its present inspection strategy to a program that is more likely to have a substantial impact on human diseases and that FSIS make such a shift as soon as possible. Further development of quantitative health risk assessment data, which must include a comprehensive evaluation of all pathogens on chickens, will be an essential tool in this change.

Whatever public health-based inspection system evolves from the risk-assessment procedure, systems for monitoring compliance with critical control point parameters and effects on product quality and public health would have to be designed. Compliance could be determined by physical measurement of contamination at critical control points and by analysis of microbial contamination, if any microbiological standards or guidelines were established. Surveillance to determine microbial contamination of the end products would provide a measure of the overall program's success in reducing the prevalence of human pathogens on market-ready poultry and would permit the tracking of trends in product contamination. Because of the influence of food handling on the occurrence of food-borne disease, however, end-product surveillance alone can not be used to judge the public health impact of the poultry inspection program. Through community-based surveillance systems (described above), FSIS could define the role of poultry products in food-borne disease in humans, establish trends to define the benefits of reduced carcass contamination, and test the relative impact of various inspection strategies.

References

Anderson, D.C., P. A. Stoesz, and A. F. Kaufmann. 1978. Psittacosis outbreak in employees of a turkey-processing plant. Am. J. Epidemiol. 107:140-148.

Anonymous. 1984. Yersiniosis today. Lancet 1:84-85.

Archer, D. L., and J. E. Kvenberg. 1985. Incidence and cost of foodborne diarrheal disease in the United States. J. Food Protect. 48:887-894.

Aserkoff, B., S. A. Schroeder, and P.S. Brachman. 1970. Salmonellosis in the United States—a five-year review. Am. J. Epidemiol. 92:13-24.

Bean, W. J., Y. Kawaoka, J. M. Wood, J. E. Pearson, and R. G. Webster. 1985. Characterization of virulent and avirulent A/chicken/ Pennsylvania/83 influenza A viruses: Potential role of defective interfering RNAs in nature. J. Virol. 54:151-160.

Biggs, P.M. 1982. The epidemiology of avian herpesviruses in veterinary medicine. Dev. Biol. Stand. 52:3-11.

Black, R. E., R. J. Jackson, T. Tsai, M. Medvesky, M. Shayegani, J. C. Feeley, K. I. E. MacLeod, and A. M. Wakelee. 1978. Epidemic Yersinia enterocolitica infection due to contaminated chocolate milk. N. Engl. J. Med. 298:76-79.

Black, R. E., M. M. Levine, M. J. Blaser, M. L. Clements, and T. P. Hughes. 1983. Studies of Campylobacter jejuni infection in volunteers. P. 13 in A. D. Pearson, M. B. Skirrow, B. Rowe, J. R. Davies, and D. M. Jones, eds. Campylobacter II: Proceedings of the Second International Workshop on Campylobacter Infections held in Brussels, September 6-9, 1983. Public Health Laboratory Service, London.

Blaser, M. J., and L. B. Reller. 1981. Campylobacter enteritis. N. Engl. J. Med. 305:1444-1452.

Blaser, M. J., J. G. Wells, R. A. Feldman, R. A. Pollard, and J. R. Allen. 1983a. Campylobacter enteritis in the United States: A multicenter study. Ann. Intern. Med. 98:360-365.

Blaser, M. J., D. N. Taylor, and R. A. Feldman. 1983b. Epidemiology of Campylobacter jejuni infections. Epidemiol. Rev. 5:157-176.

Borriella, S. P., ed. 1985. Clostridia in Gastrointestinal Disease. CRC Press, Boca Raton, Fla. 248 pp.

Bottone, E. J. 1977. Yersinia enterocolitica: A panoramic view of a charismatic microorganism. CRC Crit. Rev. Microbiol. 5:211-241.

Bottone, E. J. 1983. Current trends of Yersinia enterocolitica isolates in the New York City area. J. Clin. Microbiol. 17:63-67.

Bradbury, W. C., and D. L. G. Munroe. 1985. Occurrence of plasmids and antibiotic resistance among Campylobacter jejuni and Campylobacter coli isolated from healthy and diarrheic animals. J. Clin. Microbiol. 22:339-346.

Brouwer, R., M. J. A. Mertens, T. H. Siem, and J. Katchaki. 1979. An explosive outbreak of Campylobacter enteritis in soldiers. Antonie van Leeuwenhoek 45:517-519.

Bryan, F. L. 1980a. Foodborne diseases in the United States associated with meat and poultry. J. Food Protect. 43:140-150.

Bryan, F. L. 1980b. Poultry and poultry meat products. Pp. 410-458 in Microbial Ecology of Foods, Vol. II: Food Commodities, by the International Commission of Microbiological Specifications for Foods. Academic Press, New York.

Butzler, J.P., and M. B. Skirrow. 1979. Campylobacter enteritis. Clin. Gastroenterol. 8:737-765.

Campbell, D. F., S. S. Green, C. S. Custer, and R. W. Johnston. 1982. Incidence of Salmonella in fresh dressed turkeys raised under Salmonella-controlled and uncontrolled environments. Poult. Sci. 61:1962-1967.

Campbell, D. F., R. W. Johnston, G. S. Campbell, D. McClain, and J. F. Macaluso. 1983. The microbiology of raw, eviscerated chickens: A ten year comparison. Poult. Sci. 62:437-444.

Campbell, D. F., R. W. Johnston, M. W. Wheeler, K. V. Nagaraja, C. D. Szymansaki, and B. S. Pomeroy. 1984. Effects of the evisceration and cooling processes on the incidence of Salmonella in fresh dressed turkeys grown under Salmonella-controlled and uncontrolled environments. Poult. Sci. 63:1069-1072.

Carter, G. R. 1962. Animal serotypes of Pasteurella multocida from human infections. Can. J. Public Health 53:158-161.

Carter, G. R. 1972. Simplified identification of somatic varieties of Pasteurella multocida causing fowl cholera. Arian Dis. 16:1109-1114.

CDC (Center for Disease Control). 1977. Salmonella Surveillance, Annual Summary 1976. HEW Publ. No. (CDC) 78-8219. Center for Disease Control, Public Health Service, U.S. Department of Health, Education, and Welfare, Atlanta. 23 pp.

CDC (Center for Disease Control). 1979. Botulism in the United States, 1899-1977. Handbook for Epidemiologists, Clinicians, and Laboratory Workers. Center for Disease Control, Public Health Service, U.S. Department of Health, Education, and Welfare, Atlanta. 41 pp.

CDC (Centers for Disease Control). 1981. Salmonella Surveillance, Annual Summary 1978. HHS Publ. No. (CDC) 81-8219. Centers for Disease Control, Public Health Service, U.S. Department of Health and Human Services, Atlanta. 25 pp.

CDC (Centers for Disease Control). 1983a. Foodborne Disease Surveillance, Annual Summary 1980. HHS Publ. No. (CDC) 83-8185. Centers for Disease Control, Public Health Service, U.S. Department of Health and Human Services, Atlanta. 32 pp.

CDC (Centers for Disease Control). 1983b. Foodborne Disease Surveillance, Annual Summary 1981. HHS Publ. No. (CDC) 83-8185. Centers for Disease Control, Public Health Service, U.S. Department of Health and Human Services, Atlanta. 41 pp.

CDC (Centers for Disease Control). 1984a. Annual summary 1983: Reported morbidity and mortality in the United States. Morbid. Mortal. Weekly Rep. 32 (annual suppl.).

CDC (Centers for Disease Control). 1984b. Notifiable diseases—Reported cases by geographic division and area, United States, 1983. Morbid. Mortal. Weekly Rep. 33:542-547.

CDC (Centers for Disease Control). 1985. Foodborne Disease Surveillance, Annual Summary 1982. HHS Publ. No. (CDC) 85-8185. Centers for Disease Control, Public Health Service, U.S. Department of Health and Human Services, Atlanta. 38 pp.

CDSC (Communicable Disease Surveillance Centre). 1981. Review of Campylobacter reports to CDSC 1977-80. Communicable Dis. Rep. 12:3-4.

CEC (Commission of European Communities). 1976. Evaluation of the Hygienic Problems Related to the Chilling of Poultry Carcasses. Information on Agriculture Series No. 22. European Economic Community, Brussels. 110 pp.

Chang, P. W. 1981. Newcastle disease. Pp. 261-274 in G. W. Beran, ed. CRC Handbook Series in Zoonoses, Section B: Vital Zoonoses, Vol. II. CRC Press, Boca Raton, Fla.

Craven, P. C., W. B. Baine, D. C. Mackel, W. H. Barker, E. J. Gangarosa, M. Goldfield, H. Rosenfeld, R. Altman, G. Lachapelle, J. W. Davies, and R. C. Swanson. 1975. International outbreak of Salmonella eastbourne infection traced to contaminated chocolate. Lancet 1:788-793.

Crittenden, L. B. 1976. The epidemiology of avian lymphoid leukosis. Cancer Res. 36:570-573.

Current, W. L. 1985. Cryptosporidiosis. J. Am. Vet. Med. Assoc. 187:1334-1338.

Damsker, B., and E. J. Bottone. 1985. Mycobacterium avium-Mycobacterium intracellulare from the intestinal tracts of patients with the acquired immunodeficiency syndrome: Concepts regarding acquisition and pathogenesis. J. Infect. Dis. 151:179-181.

Dardiri, A. H., V. J. Yates, and T. D. Flanagan. 1962. The reaction to infection with the Bl strain of Newcastle disease virus in man. Am. J. Vet. Res. 23:918-921.

de Groote, G., J. Vandepitte, and G. Wauters. 1982. Surveillance of human Yersinia enterocolitica infections in Belgium: 1963-1978. J. Infect. 4:189-197.

De Wit, J. C., G. Broekhuizen, and E. H. Kampelmacher. 1979. Cross-contamination during the preparation of frozen chickens in the kitchen . J. Hyg. 83:27-32.

Durfee, P. T., M. M. Pullen, R. W. Currier II, and R. L. Parker. 1975. Human psittacosis associated with commercial processing of turkeys. J. Am. Vet. Med. Assoc. 167:804-808.

Faddoul, G. P., and G. W. Fellows. 1966. A five-year survey of the incidence of salmonellae in avian species. Arian Dis. 10:296-304.

Fagerberg, D. J., and C. L. Quarles. 1982. Final Report, Phases I, II, III, 1978-1981. Data Base for Drug Resistant Bacteria for Animals. Prepared for the U.S. Food and Drug Administration. FDA Contract No. 223-77-7032. Animal Sciences Department, Colorado State University, Fort Collins, Colo. [1590 pp.]

Fenner, F., B. R. McAuslan, C. A. Mims, J. Sambrook, and D. O. White. 1974. Viral oncogenesis: RNA viruses. Pp. 508-542 in The Biology of Animal Viruses, 2nd ed. Academic Press, New York.

Filstein, M. R., A. B. Ley, M. S. Vernon, K. A. Gaffney, and L. T. Glickman. 1981. Epidemic of psittacosis in a college of veterinary medicine . J. Am. Vet. Med. Assoc. 179:569-574.

Finch, M. J., and L. W. Riley. 1984. Campylobacter infections in the United States: Results of an 11-state surveillance. Arch. Intern. Med. 144:1610-1612.

Gangarosa, E. J. 1978a. Epidemiology of Escherichia coli in the United States. J. Infect. Dis. 137:634-638.

Gangarosa, E. J. 1978b. What have we learned from 15 years of Salmonella surveillance? Pp. 9-28 in the Proceedings of the National Salmonellosis Seminar held in Washington, D.C., January 10-11, 1978. U.S. Animal Health Association, Richmond, Va.

Gangarosa, E. J., and M. H. Merson. 1977. Epidemiologic assessment of the relevance of the so-called enteropathogenic serogroups of Escherichia coli in diarrhea. N. Engl. J. Med. 296:1210-1213.

Gemski, P., J. R. Lazere, and T. Casey. 1980. Plasmid associated with pathogenicity and calcium dependency of Yersinia enterocolitica . Infect. Immun. 27:682-685.

Ghosh, A. C. 1978. Prevalence of Bacillus cereus in the faeces of healthy adults. J. Hyg. 80:233-236.

Gilbert, R. J. 1979. Bacillus cereus gastroenteritis. Pp. 495-518 in H. Riemann and F. L. Bryan, eds. Food-borne Infections and Intoxications, 2nd ed. Academic Press, New York.

Gilbert, R. J., and J. M. Parry. 1977. Serotypes of Bacillus cereus from outbreaks of food poisoning and from routine foods. J. Hyg. 78:69-74.

Gilbert, R. J., M. F. Stringer, and T. C. Peace. 1974. The survival and growth of Bacillus cereus in boiled and fried rice in relation to outbreaks of food poisoning. J. Hyg. 73:433-444.

Glantz, P. J. 1971. Serotypes of Escherichia coli associated with colibacillosis in neonatal animals. Ann. N.Y. Acad. Sci. 176:67-79.

Goepfert, J. M., W. M. Spira, and H. U. Kim. 1972. Bacillus cereus : Food poisoning organism. A review. J. Milk Food Technol. 35:213-227.

Good, R. C. 1985. Opportunistic pathogens in the genus Mycobacterium . Annu. Rev. Microbiol. 39:347-369.

Grant, I. H., N. J. Richardson, and V. D. Bokkenheuser. 1980. Broiler chickens as potential sources of Campylobacter infections in humans. J. Clin. Microbiol. 11:508-510.

Green, S. S., A. B. Moran, R. W. Johnston, P. Uhler, and J. Chiu. 1982. The incidence of Salmonella species and serotypes in young whole chicken carcasses in 1979 as compared with 1967. Poult. Sci. 61:288-293.

Gross, R. J. 1983. Escherichia coli diarrhoea. J. Infect. 7:177-192.

Guerrant, R. L. 1980. Yet another pathogenic mechanism for Escherichia coli diarrhea. N. Engl. J. Med. 302:113-115.

Hariharan, H., and W. R. Mitchell. 1977. Type C botulism: The agent, host spectrum and environment. Vet. Bull. 47:95-103.

Harris, N. V., N. S. Weiss, and C. M. Nolan. 1986a. The role of poultry and meats in the etiology of Campylobacter jejuni/coli enteritis. Am. J. Public Health 76:407-411.

Harris, N. V., D. Thompson, D.C. Martin, and C. M. Nolan. 1986b. A survey of Campylobacter and other bacterial contaminants of pre-market chicken and retail poultry and meats, King County, Washington. Am. J. Public Health 76:401-406.

Hauge, S. 1950. Matforgiftninger fremkalt av Bacillus cereus. Nord. Hyg. Tidskr. 31:189-206.

Hauge, S. 1955. Food poisoning caused by aerobic spore-forming bacilli. J. Appl. Bacteriol. 18:591-595.

Hauschild, A. H. W., and F. L. Bryan. 1980. Estimate of cases of food and waterborne illness in Canada and the United States. J. Food Protect. 43:435-440, 446.

Hayflick, L., ed. 1969. The Mycoplasmatales and the L-Phase of Bacteria. Appleton-Century-Crofts, New York. 750 pp.

Heesemann, J., B. Algermissen, and R. Laufs. 1984. Genetically manipulated virulence of Yersinia enterocolitica. Infect. Immun. 46:105-110.

Hehlmann, R., D. Kufe, and S. Spiegelman. 1972. Viral-related RNA in Hodgkins' disease and other human lymphomas. Proc. Natl. Acad. Sci. U.S.A. 69:1727-1731.

Helmuth, R., R. Stephan, C. Bunge, B. Hoog, A. Steinbeck, and E. Bulling. 1985. Epidemiology of virulence-associated plasmids and outer membrane protein patterns within seven common Salmonella serotypes. Infect. Immun. 48:175-182.

Hines, M. P., P. M. Page, N. Hirschberg, and L. G. Maddry. 1957. Ornithosis and leptospirosis survey of a chicken and turkey processing plant and textile mill in North Carolina. Vet. Med. 52:337-338, 356.

Hook, E. W. 1985. Salmonella species (including typhoid fever). Pp. 1256-1269 in G. L. Mandell, R. G. Douglas, Jr., and J. E. Bennett, eds. Principles and Practice of Infectious Diseases, 2nd ed. Wiley, New York.

Hopkins, R. S., and A. S. Scott. 1983. Handling raw chicken as a source for sporadic Campylobacter jejuni infections. J. Infect. Dis. 148:770.

Hornick, R. B. 1983. Nontyphoidal salmonellosis. Pp. 655-661 in P. D. Hoeprich , ed. Infectious Diseases: A Modern Treatise of Infectious Processes, 3rd ed. Harper & Row, Philadelphia.

Horwitz, M. A., and E. J. Gangarosa. 1976. Foodborne disease outbreaks traced to poultry, United States, 1966-1974. J. Milk Food Technol. 39:859-863.

Hughes, J. M., J. R. Blumenthal, M. H. Merson, G. L. Lombard, V. R. Dowell, and E. J. Gangarosa. 1981. Clinical features of type-A and type-B food-borne botulism. Ann. Intern. Med. 95:442-445.

Hutchinson, D. N., H. C. Dawkins, and F. J. Bolton. 1983. Do campylobacters contaminate food preparation areas? Pp. 169-170 in A. D. Pearson, M. B. Skirrow, B. Rowe, J. R. Davies, and D. M. Jones, eds. Campylobacter II: Proceedings of the Second International Workshop on Campylobacter Infections held in Brussels, September 6-9, 1983. Public Health Laboratory Service, London.

Hyams, J. S., W. A. Durbin, R. J. Grand, and D. A. Goldmann. 1980. Salmonella bacteremia in the first year of life. J. Pediatr. 96:57-59.

Inoue, Y. K. 1973. Arian infectious laryngotracheitis and S.M.O.N. in Japan. Lancet 1:1009.

Inoue, Y. 1975. An avian-related new herpesvirus infection in man—subacute myelo-optico-neuropathy (SMON). Prog. Med. Virol. 21:32-42.

Inoue, Y. K., and Y. Nishibe. 1973. Serological relationship between S.M.O.N. virus and avian infectious laryngotracheitis virus. Lancet 1:776-777.

Ionescu, G., C. Ienistea, and C. Ionescu. 1966. Freeventa B. cereus in laptele crud si in laptele pasteurizat. Microbiol., Parazitol., Epidemiol. 11:423-430.

Kaplan, M. M. 1980. Some epidemiological and virological relationships between human and animal influenza. Comp. Immunol. Microbiol. Infect. Dis. 3:19-24.

Kay, B. A., K. Wachsmuth, P. Gemski, J. C. Feeley, T. J. Quan, and D. J. Brenner. 1983. Virulence and phenotypic characterization of Yersinia enterocolitica isolated from humans in the United States. J. Clin. Microbiol. 17:128-138.

Kendall, E. J. C., and E. I. Tanner. 1982. Campylobacter enteritis in general practice. J. Hyg. 88:155-163.

Kinde, H., C. A. Genigeorgis, and M. Pappaioanou. 1983. Prevalence of Campylobacter jejuni in chicken wings. Appl. Environ. Microbiol. 45:1116-1118.

Kist, M. 1983. Campylobacter enteritis in an industrial country' Epidemiologic features in urban and rural areas. P. 140 in A. D. Pearson, M. B. Skirrow, B. Rowe, J. R. Davies, and D. M. Jones, eds. Campylobacter II: Proceedings of the Second International Workshop on Campylobacter Infections held in Brussels, September 6-9, 1983. Public Health Laboratory Service, London.

Klipstein, F. A., R. F. Engert, H. Short, and E. A. Schenk. 1985. Pathogenic properties of Campylobacter jejuni: Assay and correlation with clinical manifestations. Infect. Immun. 50:43-49.

Kuritsky, J. N., G. P. Schmid, M. E. Potter, D.C. Anderson, and A. F. Kaufmann. 1984. Psittacosis—a diagnostic challenge. J. Occup. Med. 26:731-733.

Larsen, J. H. 1980. Yersinia enterocolitica infections and rheumatic diseases. Scand. J. Rheumatol. 9:129-137.

Lee, W. H. 1977. An assessment of Yersinia enterocolitica and its presence in foods. J. Food Protect. 40:486-489.

Levine, M. M. 1985. Escherichia coli infections. N. Engl. J. Med. 313:445-447.

Linton, A. H., ed. 1983. Guidelines on Prevention and Control of Salmonellosis. World Health Organization, Geneva. 128 pp.

MacCready, R. A., J.P. Reardon, and I. Saphra. 1957. Salmonellosis in Massachusetts; a sixteen-year experience. N. Engl. J. Med. 256:1121-1128.

Makari, J. G. 1973. Association between Marek's herpesvirus and human cancer. I. Detection of cross-reacting antigens between chicken tumors and human tumors. Oncology 28:177-183.

Mandal, B. K., and V. Mani. 1976. Colonic involvement in salmonellosis. Lancet 1:887-888.

Marks, M. I., C. H. Pal, L. Lafleur, L. Lackman, and O. Hammerberg. 1980. Yersinia enterocolitica gastroenteritis: A prospective study of clinical, bacteriologic, and epidemiologic features. J. Pediatr. 96:26-31.

Marymont, J. H., Jr., K. K. Durfee, H. Alexander, and J.P. Smith. 1982. Yersinia enterocolitica in Kansas: Attempted recovery from 1,212 patients. Am. J. Clin. Pathol. 77:753-755.

Mathan, V. I., D. P. Rajah, F. A. Klipstein, and R. F. Engert. 1984. Enterotoxigenic Campylobacter jejuni among children in South India. Lancet 2:981.

McCullough, N. B., and C. W. Eisele. 1951. Experimental human salmonellosis; pathogenicity of strains of Salmonella newport, Salmonella derby and Salmonella bareilly obtained from spray-dried whole egg. J. Infect. Dis. 89:209-213.

McGaughey, C. A. 1932. Organisms of the B. influenzae group in fowls. J. Comp. Pathol. Ther. 45:58-66.

Meissner, G., and W. Ariz. 1977. Sources of Mycobacterium avium complex infection resulting in human diseases. Am. Rev. Respir. Dis. 116:1057-1064.

Meyer, K. F., and B. Eddie. 1942. Spontaneous ornithosis (psittacosis) in chickens the cause of a human infection. Proc. Soc. Exp. Biol. Med. 49:522-525.

Midura, T., M. Gerber, R. Wood, and A. R. Leonard. 1970. Outbreak of food poisoning caused by Bacillus cereus. Public Health Rep. 85:45-48.

Miller, L. T., and V. J. Yates. 1971. Reactions of human sera to avian adenoviruaes and Newcastle disease virus. Arian Dis. 15:781-788.

Morris, G. K., and J. C. Feeley. 1976. Yersinia enterocolitica: A review of its role in food hygiene. Bull. W.H.O. 54:79-85.

Morris, J. G., Jr. 1981. Bacillus cereus food poisoning. Arch. Intern. Med. 141:711.

Morris, J. G., Jr., and R. E. Black. 1985. Cholera and other vibrioses in the United States. N. Engl. J. Med. 312:343-350.

Morris, J. G., Jr., and C. L. Hatheway. 1983. Botulism. Pp. 1115-1124 in P. D. Hoeprich, ed. Infectious Diseases: A Modern Treatise of Infectious Processes, 3rd ed. Harper & Row, Philadelphia.

Murphy, B. R., and R. G. Webster. 1985. Influenza viruses. Pp. 1179-1239 in B. N. Fields, D. M. Knipe, R. M. Chanock, J. L. Melnick, B. Roizman, and R. E. Shope, eds. Virology. Raven Press, New York.

Naito, M., K. Oho, S. Tanabe, T. Doi, and S. Kato. 1970. Detection in chicken and human sera of antibody against herpes type virus from a chicken with Marek's disease and EB virus demonstrated by the indirect immunofluorescence test. Biken J. 13:205-212.

Navin, T. R. 1985. Cryptosporidiosis in humans: Review of recent epidemiologic studies. Eur. J. Epidemiol. 1:77-83.

Nerome, K., Y. Yoshioka, C. A. Torres, A. Oya, P. Bachmann, K. Ottis, and R. G. Webster. 1984. Persistence of Q strain of H2N2 influenza virus in avian species: Antigenic, biological and genetic analysis of avian and human H2N2 viruses. Arch. Virol. 81:239-250.

Nishimura, C., and T. Tobe. 1973. Antigenicity of S.M.O.N.-associated virus closely related to avian infectious laryngotracheitis virus. Lancet 2:1445.

Norkrans, G., and A. Svedham. 1982. Epidemiological aspects of Campylobacter jejuni enteritis. J. Hyg. 89:163-170.

NRC (National Research Council). 1969. An Evaluation of the Salmonella Problem. Report of the Committee on Salmonella, Division of Biology and Agriculture. National Academy of Sciences, Washington, D.C. 207 pp.

NRC (National Research Council). 1985a. An Evaluation of the Role of Microbiological Criteria in Foods and Food Ingredients. Report of the Subcommittee on Microbiological Criteria, Committee on Food Protection, Food and Nutrition Board. National Academy Press, Washington, D.C. 436 pp.

NRC (National Research Council). 1985b. Meat and Poultry Inspection: The Scientific Basis of the Nation's Program. Report of the Committee on the Scientific Basis of the Nation's Meat and Poultry Inspection Program, Food and Nutrition Board. National Academy Press, Washington, D.C. 209 pp.

Nygren, B. 1962. Phospholipase C-producing bacteria and food poisoning. An experimental study on Clostridium perfringens and Bacillus cereus. Acta Pathol. Microbiol. Scand., Suppl. 160:1-88.

Pai, C. H., S. Sorger, L. Lackman, R. E. Sinai, and M. I. Marks. 1979. Campylobacter gastroenteritis in children. J. Pediatr. 94:589-591.

Portnoy, D. A., S. L. Moseley, and S. Falkow. 1981. Characterization of plasmids and plasmid-associated determinants of Yersinia enterocolitica pathogenesis. Infect. Immun. 31:775-782.

Potter, M. E., and A. F. Kaufmann. 1979. Psittacosis in humans in the United States, 1975-1977. J. Infect. Dis. 140:131-134.

Purchase, H. G., and R. L. Witter. 1986. Public health concerns from human exposure to oncogenic avian herpesviruses. J. Am. Vet. Med. Assoc. 189:1430-1436.

Reagan, R. L., S. C. Chang, F. S. Yancey, and A. L. Brueckner. 1956. Isolation of Newcastle disease virus from man with confirmation by electron microscopy. J. Am. Vet. Med. Assoc. 129:79-80.

Rechtman, J., L. Lapeyrie, and H. H. Mollaret. 1985. Contribution à l'écologie de Yersinia enterocolitica et espèces apparentées: Recherche dans des denrées alimentaires . Med. Mal. Infect. 15:130-134.

Richman, A. V., C. G. Aulisio, W. G. Jahnes, and N. M. Tauraso. 1972. Arian leukosis antibody response in individuals given chicken embryo derived vaccines. Proc. Soc. Exp. Biol. Med. 139:235-237.

Riley, L. W., and M. J. Finch. 1985. Results of the first year of national surveillance of Campylobacter infections in the United States. J. Infect. Dis. 151:956-959.

Roizman, B., and W. Batterson. 1985. Herpesviruses and their replication. Pp. 497-525 in B. N. Fields, D. M. Knipe, R. M. Chanock, J. L. Melnick, B. Roizman, and R. E. Shope, eds. Virology. Raven Press, New York.

Rosenberg, M. L., E. J. Gangarosa, R. A. Pollard, O. Brolnitsky, and J. S. Marr. 1977. Shigella surveillance in the United States, 1975. J. Infect. Dis. 136:458-460.

Roth, F. K., and R. M. Dougherty. 1971. Search for group-specific antibodies of avian leukosis virus in human leukemic sera. J. Natl. Cancer Inst. 46:1357-1359.

Ruiz-Palacios, G. M., J. Torres, N. I. Torres, E. Escamilla, B. R. Ruiz-Palacios, and J. Tamayo. 1983. Cholera-like enterotoxin produced by Campylobacter jejuni. Lancet 2:250-253.

Saphra, I., and M. Wassermann. 1954. Salmonella cholerae suis: A clinical and epidemiological evaluation of 329 infections identified between 1940 and 1954 in the New York Salmonella Center. Am. J. Med. Sci. 228:525-533.

Schaefer, W. B. 1968. Incidence of the serotypes of Mycobacterium avium and atypical mycobacteria in human and animal diseases. Am. Rev. Respir. Dis. 97:18-23.

Schiemann, D. A., and J. A. Devenish. 1982. Relationship of HeLa cell infectivity to biochemical, serological, and virulence characteristics of Yersinia enterocolitica. Infect. Immun. 35:497-506.

Schiemann, D. A., and S. Toma. 1978. Isolation of Yersinia enterocolitica from raw milk. Appl. Environ. Microbiol. 35:54-58.

Scott, A. B. 1981. Botulinum toxin injection of eye muscles to correct strabismus. Trans. Am. Ophthalmol. Soc. 79:734-770.

Serény, B. 1955. Experimental Shigella keratoconjunctivitis; a preliminary report. Acta Microbiol. Acad. Sci. Hung. 2:293-296.

Sharma, J. M., R. L. Witter, B. R. Burmester, and J. C. Landon. 1973. Public health implications of Marek's disease virus and herpesvirus of turkeys. Studies on human and subhuman primates. J. Natl. Cancer Inst. 51:1123-1128.

Shayegani, M., D. Morse, I. DeForge, T. Root, L. M. Parsons, and P.S. Maupin. 1983. Microbiology of a major foodborne outbreak of gastroenteritis caused by Yersinia enterocolitica serogroup 0:8. J. Clin. Microbiol. 17:35-40.

Silverstolpe, L., U. Plazikowski, J. Kjellander, and G. Vahlne. 1961. An epidemic among infants caused by Salmonella muenchen. J. Appl. Bacteriol. 24:134-142.

SKCDPH (Seattle-King County Department of Public Health). 1984. Surveillance of the Flow of Salmonella and Campylobacter in a Community. Prepared for the Bureau of Veterinary Medicine, U.S. Food and Drug Administration. Contract No. 223-81-7041. Communicable Disease Control Section, Seattle-King County Department of Public Health, Seattle. [250 pp.]

Skirrow, M. B. 1977. Campylobacter enteritis: A "new" disease. Br. Med. J. 2:9-11.

Smith, J. E. 1955. Studies on Pasteurella septica. I. The occurrence in the nose and tonsils of dogs. J. Comp. Pathol. 65:239-245.

Smitherman, R. E., C. A. Genigeorgis, and T. B. Farver. 1984. Preliminary observations on the occurrence of Campylobacter jejuni at four California chicken ranches. J. Food Protect. 47:293-298.

Snyder, J. D., E. Christenson, and R. A. Feldman. 1982. Human Yersinia enterocolitica infections in Wisconsin: Clinical, laboratory and epidemiologic features. Am. J. Med. 72:768-774.

Solomon J. J., and H. G. Purchase. 1969. A search for avian leukosis virus and antiviral activity in the blood of leukemic and nonleukemic adults and children. J. Natl. Cancer Inst. 42:29-33.

Sours, H. E., and D. G. Smith. 1980. Outbreaks of foodborne disease in the United States, 1972-1978. J. Infect. Dis. 142:122-125.

Stengel, G. 1985. Yersinia enterocolitica. Occurrence and importance in foods. Fleischwirtschaft 65:1493-1495.

Stern, N. J., S. S. Green, N. Thaker, D. J. Krout, and J. Chiu. 1984. Recovery of Campylobacter jejuni from fresh and frozen meat and poultry collected at slaughter. J. Food Protect. 47:372-374.

Surkiewicz, B. F., R. W. Johnston, A. B. Moran, and G. W. Krumm. 1969. A bacteriological survey of chicken eviscerating plants. Food Technol. 23:1066-1069.

Szita, J., M. Kali, and B. Rédey. 1973. Incidence of Yersinia enterocolitica infection in Hungary. Pp. 106-110 in A. Grumbach, ed. Contributions to Microbiology and Immunology, Vol. 2. Karger, New York.

Tacket, C. O., J. Ballard, N. Harris, J. Allard, C. Nolan, T. Quan, and M. L. Cohen. 1985. An outbreak of Yersinia enterocolitica infections caused by contaminated tofu (soybean curd). Am. J. Epidemiol. 121:705-711.

Terranova, W., and P. A. Blake. 1978. Bacillus cereus food poisoning. N. Engl. J. Med. 298:143-144.

Thoen, C. O., A. G. Karlson, and E. M. Himes. 1981. Mycobacterial infections in animals. Rev. Infect. Dis. 3:960-972.

Todd, E. C. D. 1980. Poultry-associated foodborne disease—its occurrence, cost, sources and prevention. J. Food Protect. 43:129-139.

Turnbull, P. C. B., T. A. French, and E. G. Dowsett. 1977. Severe systemic and pyogenic infections with Bacillus cereus. Br. Med. J. 1:1628-1629.

Turnbull, P. C. B., K. Jorgensen, J. M. Kramer, R. J. Gilbert, and J. M. Parry. 1979. Severe clinical conditions associated with <u>Bacillus cereus</u> and the apparent involvement of exotoxins. J. Clin. Pathol. 32:289-293.

Vantrappen, G., K. Geboes, and E. Ponette. 1982. Yersinia enteritis. Med. Clin. North Am. 66:639-653.

Walter, S. D. 1975. The distribution of Levin's measure of attributable risk. Biometrika 62:371-374.

Waters, T. D., P.S. Anderson, Jr., G. W. Beebe, and R. W. Miller. 1972. Yellow fever vaccination, avian leukosis virus, and cancer risk in man. Science 177:76-77.

Wempe, J. M., C. A. Genigeorgis, T. B. Farver, and H. I. Yusufu. 1983. Prevalence of <u>Campylobacter jejuni</u> in two California chicken processing plants. Appl. Environ. Microbiol. 45:355-359.

Wolinsky, E. 1979. Nontuberculous mycobacteria and associated diseases. Am. Rev. Respir. Dis. 119:107-159.

Wood, J. M., R. G. Webster, and V. F. Nettles. 1985. Host range of A/chicken/Pennsylvania/83 (H5N2) influenza virus. Arian Dis. 29:198-207.

Chapter 5

Application of the Model to Chemical Hazards

The Committee on the Scientific Basis of the Nation's Meat and Poultry Inspection Program (NRC, 1985) described the various sources of chemical residues in meat and poultry products and the approach used by FSIS to control them. That committee also made several recommendations for improving the FSIS inspection program and urged the adoption of formal risk-assessment procedures to provide maximum protection of public health. Specifically, the committee recommended that risk assessment play a major role in the establishment of limits for chemical residues in meat and poultry products destined for human consumption, in the prevention and characterization of hazards, in the setting of priorities for controlling residues, and in the design of sampling methods. This chapter contains a discussion of risk assessment as a guide to the management of chemical hazards in poultry products, criteria for judging the safety of poultry products containing residues, some approaches to ensuring that safety criteria are met, and the types of data and analysis needed to assess the public health impact of chemical residues in poultry products. It also identifies the necessary elements of a risk-management program and describes the risk-assessment methods needed to establish this program. It does not include consideration of current FSIS inspection, which is evaluated in subsequent chapters of the report.

GENERAL METHODS FOR ASSESSING THE PUBLIC HEALTH RISKS OF CHEMICALS

There is extensive documentation on deaths and injuries from accidental poisonings by household products, pesticides, and therapeutic agents. Ordinarily there is little difficulty in estimating the relationship between the extent to which these substances are used and the frequency of poisonings and in documenting the association between a given exposure and a given poisoning when the effect is immediately observable (i.e., acute). It is more difficult to assess risks associated with chemical exposures when no immediately observable effects are produced when the fact or degree of exposure is itself highly uncertain. Since most chemical exposures associated with residues in poultry products are uncertain, the risks must be predicted and those predictions used to set health protection standards.

Although the methods used to predict chemical risks are uncertain (e.g., because of incomplete data, the need to extrapolate beyond data, and the lack of knowledge concerning the extent of future human exposure), they are based on a strong scientific foundation (NRC, 1980b, 1983). The safe use of products, including food ingredients, pesticides, and drugs, depends upon these methods of risk prediction and their use in the establishment of low risk (or safe) exposures (FSC, 1980).

People are exposed to a large number of naturally occurring and man-made chemicals through poultry products and other environmental media. If they are to be protected from the possible adverse effects of these substances, methods to assess the risk assessment of such exposures must be applied. It is a premise of this report that predictive methods developed for and widely used in many areas of public health protection are appropriate for assessing the risks of exposure to chemical residues, establishing appropriate health protection standards for such residues, and guiding the development of programs to manage the risks presented by the residues. Parts or all of this premise have been adopted by the Food and Drug Administration, the Environmental Protection Agency, and other government agencies charged with protecting consumers from such residues, especially for risk assessment and the establishment of standards. However, there are important limitations in the methods themselves and in their application to specific problems, including those associated with poultry products.

THE COMPONENTS OF RISK ASSESSMENT

A National Research Council committee described four basic components of risk assessment in the federal government: hazard identification, dose-response assessment, exposure assessment, and risk characterization (NRC, 1983). Figure 5-1 shows the relationships between these components of risk assessment, research, and risk management.

Hazard Identification

Toxicity. All chemical substances, whether natural or man-made, can cause some form of biological injury under some conditions of exposure. The purpose of the first phase of risk assessment is to collect and evaluate information on the inherent toxic properties of chemicals of interest. Identifying these properties is not equivalent to identifying possible risk. Thus, it should not be assumed that a substance displaying toxicity presents a risk to human health. All steps of risk assessment must be completed before any statement can be made about risk.

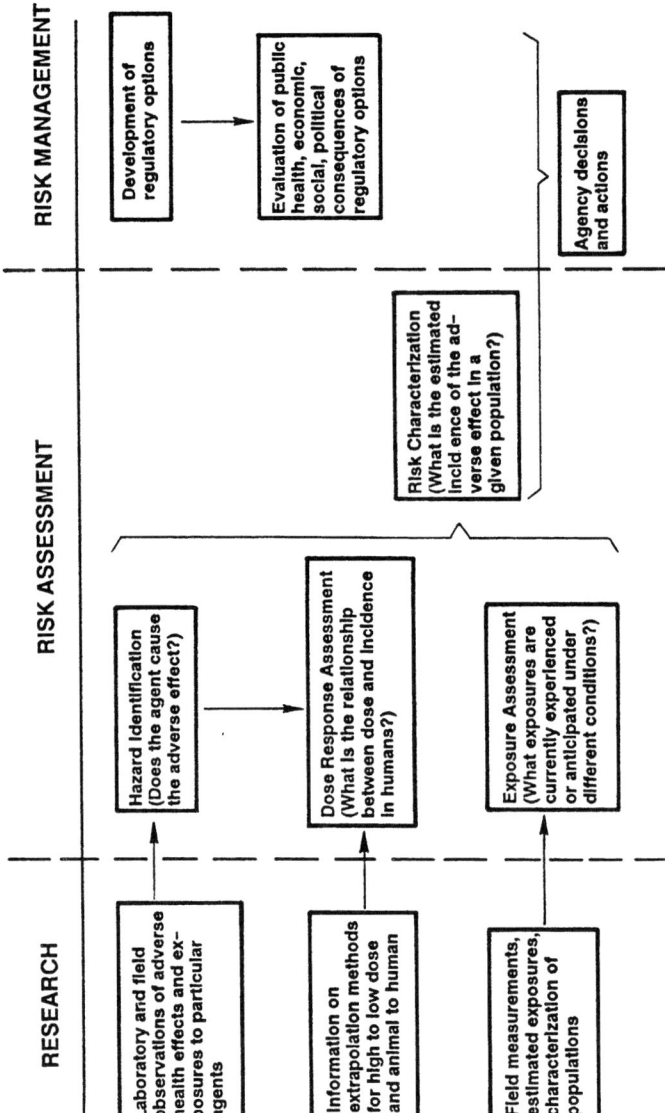

Figure 5-1
Elements of risk assessment and risk management. From NRC, 1984.

There are two principal sources of information about the toxic properties of chemical substances: investigations of exposed human populations or individuals (epidemiological or clinical investigations) and experimental studies in laboratory animals or other biological systems. Knowledge of the molecular structure of some substances may be helpful in predicting toxic properties, but this aspect of toxicological science is still immature (Asher and Zervos, 1977; Klaassen and Doull, 1980; NRC, 1980b; OSTP, 1985).

Data on Humans. Well-conducted epidemiological and clinical investigations provide pertinent data for the evaluation of the hazardous properties of environmental agents. Epidemiological studies have provided convincing evidence about the cancer-causing properties of such agents as cigarette smoke, asbestos, vinyl chloride, and diethylstilbestrol (DES) and about the teratogenic effect of thalidomide. Clinical investigations of exposed persons have provided information on the toxicity of consumer and industrial products (MacMahon and Pugh, 1970; OSTP, 1985). There are, however, the following limitations in the use of both epidemiological and clinical data for identifying the toxic properties of chemical substances:

- The deliberate, controlled exposure of human beings to identify toxic effects is, with few exceptions, unethical. Exceptions include short-term exposures to substances (e.g., certain drugs) that produce mild, fully reversible effects.
- Epidemiological and clinical studies cannot be conducted on newly introduced chemicals or chemicals for which there has been little or no previous human exposure.
- Accurate data on the chemical nature of the substances to which populations or individuals may have been exposed and on the intensity and duration of their exposure are rarely available, especially when exposures have taken place in the distant past.
- It is difficult to provide proper controls for epidemiological studies when the cause-and-effect relationships of a chemical cannot be easily established, as is the case for chemical workers who maybe exposed to unknown amounts of other substances in addition to the chemical of immediate interest.
- In investigations of diseases with long latent periods, such as cancer, it is usually difficult to follow exposed persons for periods long enough for the disease to reach a clinically detectable state and thus for firm conclusions to be drawn about the presence or absence of an effect.
- Epidemiological studies cannot generally detect small but possibly important changes unless the study population is very large (rarely practicable) or the resulting disease is rare (e.g., occurrence of vaginal adenocarcinoma during adolesence in daughters of mothers given DES during pregnancy).

Because of these limitations, public health officials must frequently turn to experimental data for information about the toxic properties of chemicals in the environment.

Experimental Animal Data. Laboratory animal studies have an advantage over epidemiological and clinical investigations (NRC, 1980b). The experiments can be controlled so that causal relationships between exposure to a substance and toxicity can be established, and the relationship between the intensity and duration of exposure and the magnitude of toxicity can be studied (NRC, 1980b). (See section on Dose-Response Assessment below.) Animals can be studied for functional changes or killed at various times during the experiment and examined for the presence of a variety of biological injuries and pathological changes that are not observable clinically. In rats and mice, the effects of lifetime exposures to an agent can be detected in 2 or 3 years—the normal lifespan of these species (OSTP, 1985).

These advantages of data from animal studies are partially offset by the obvious fact that animals are not biologically identical to humans. To conclude that some agent can cause a certain form of toxicity in humans because it does so in laboratory animals requires inclusion of some untested assumptions about the biological similarity of various mammalian species. There is evidence that results from animal studies are often applicable to humans. For example, most substances known to be carcinogenic in humans are also carcinogenic in animals. Similar examples could be collected for a variety of other toxic effects (NRC, 1983; OSTP, 1985). Exceptions are also common, however.

Unless human data are adequate to refute a specific finding of toxicity in animals or there is some other biological reason to do so, it is reasonable to infer a potential for toxicity in humans from observations in experimental studies of animals. Animal experiments are the principal source of toxicity data for assessing the human risks and safety of pesticides, food and color additives, and food and drinking water contaminants, and there is no reason not to rely on such data for similar assessments of chemical residues in poultry products.

Manifestations of Toxicity and Tests to Identify Them. Systematic investigation of the toxicity of a chemical substance usually begins with a determination of its acute toxicity, which includes a determination of the dose of a substance that in a single exposure (lethal dose) will cause the deaths of the exposed animals within a short time after administration. At successively lower levels of exposure, the percentage of animals that respond decreases correspondingly. The relationship between dose and the percentage of the animal population that dies is called the dose-response relationship for the end point in question—in this case, death. The range of doses over which deaths are observed and the shape of the dose-response relationship vary from one substance to another, and both are critical to an assessment of a substance's capacity to cause death in an exposed population.

Short-term exposures (i.e., one or several exposures repeated over several days or a few weeks) to chemical substances in amounts lower than the lethal dose may produce toxicity that ranges from mild (e.g., reversible eye or skin irritation or transitory nervous system disorders) to severe (e.g., irreversible blindness or liver damage). The toxic manifestations of a short-term exposure to a chemical depend on the intensity and duration of the exposure and the characteristics of the chemicals (Doull et al., 1980; Loomis, 1978; NRC, 1983).

Studies of short-term exposures are generally followed by studies of long-term exposures to lower doses (chronic toxicity) (NRC, 1980b). These experiments are designed to detect effects that arise after many repeated, sometimes daily, exposures that occur over various periods—from approximately 10% of an animal's lifespan (subchronic toxicity studies) to its full lifespan (2-3 years for rodents; several times longer for other commonly used animals such as dogs and monkeys) or effects resulting from short-term exposures that do not become clinically detectable until much later (e.g., for DES). Chronic effects may range from relatively mild conditions to progressive and lethal lesions such as cancer. The form of injury or disease and its dose-response characteristics are specific to the chemical, but both these features of chemical toxicity can be altered by characteristics of the exposed animal (e.g., its genetic background, health status, age, or sex) and its environment (e.g., the nature of its diet or the presence of other environmental agents). Such interspecies and intraspecies differences in toxic response and dose-response characteristics for a given substance have strongly influenced the methods used by public health scientists to assess risks. (See section on Risk Characterization below).

Subchronic toxicity experiments can reveal much about the potential of a substance to injure various organs and systems of the body, including the developing fetus, but they cannot reveal whether a substance can induce cancer (OSTP, 1985), except when it is unusually potent. Determination of carcinogenicity usually requires that test animals be exposed for most of their lifetimes.

There are now many well-validated test systems used worldwide by both public health agencies and private concerns to establish the acute, subchronic, and chronic toxicities of chemical substances (EPA, 1982; FDA, 1982b; NRC, 1977). The most thoroughly tested substances are those that must, by law, be evaluated before they can be introduced into commerce (e.g., food and color additives, drugs, and pesticides) (NRC, 1985).

Quality and Extent of Data. The quantity and quality of toxicity data available on different substances vary greatly. For a few substances the data base may be extensive and may include results of all the standard toxicity tests as well as data specific to each substance under evaluation, whereas for other substances, the data base may include, at best, only a determination of acute toxicity or no significant toxicity data at all. For most important industrial chemicals, the quantity and quality of available data fall somewhere between these two extremes, but more toward the lower end of the scale (NPC, 1984).

There is no straightforward way to define the adequacy of a given data base. A data base may be sufficient to determine the safety of a certain use or type of chemical exposure but may be inadequate to determine the risk presented by another use or type of exposure. For example, many agents tested for occupational risk have not been examined for their potential to cause chronic toxicity or birth defects. If such substances show up in the poultry supply because of environmental pollution, the absence of information on chronic effects and their effect on the developing fetus would be of great concern. Similarly, the absence of chronic toxicity data on many chemicals is of concern if the chemicals are found to be present in poultry products to which people could be chronically exposed. The absence of data does not imply that a risk exists, but it does mean that risk (and therefore safety) cannot be ascertained with an adequate degree of confidence. Various methods are used to compensate for such data gaps. These methods are described below in the section on Risk Characterization.

Hazard Evaluation. This phase of risk assessment includes a critical review of clinical, epidemiological, and experimental toxicity data and identification of the inherent hazardous properties of a substance, the degree to which these hazards are known, and the uncertainties in the data. A critical feature of this process are judgments about the strength of inferences for human risk from data derived from animal studies. At this stage of risk assessment, no attempt is made to determine the degree of human risk that might be associated with the substance under evaluation.

Dose-Response Assessment

For an exposure of a given duration, the frequency and severity of toxic effects in an exposed population (the risk) generally increase with increasing dose. Toxic effects may also change as exposure increases. The dose-response relationship is critical to risk assessment and must therefore be well defined. Well-defined dose-response relationships can rarely be obtained from epidemiological studies because of uncertainty regarding the exposures that produced the toxic responses seen. Therefore, experimental data are the primary sources of dose-response information for risk assessment.

The dose of a toxic agent can be expressed in various ways. Most commonly it is presented as the weight (mg) of the agent taken into the body per unit (kg) of body weight (mg) of the human or test animal per unit of time (usually, per day), e.g., mg/kg bw/day. Dividing intake by body weight permits comparisons to be made among species with different average body weights. Other measures of dose, such as mg/kg bw over a lifetime, mg/m^2 of body surface area, parts per million (ppm) in air, water, or diet, are used less often.

For most toxic effects, a threshold dose is the amount of exposure that must be exceeded before a specific toxic effect is produced. For other effects such as cancer, however, there appears to be a biological basis for rejecting the threshold hypothesis. As currently practiced, in fact, carcinogenic risk assessment is generally based on the assumption that there is no threshold dose. Rather than entering more fully into the complex debate on thresholds, the committee has simply adopted the positions taken by the major regulatory and public health agencies and other NRC committees, i.e., the absence of a threshold for carcinogens.

A critical part of dose-response assessment is identification of the dose that produces no adverse response, i.e., the no-observed-effect level (NOEL), in the treated animals. The NOEL is generally taken as the starting point for risk assessment of virtually all effects other than cancer. It may approximate a threshold dose for the animal population under study, but for a variety of reasons the experimentally determined NOEL is probably not identical to the true threshold dose.

For carcinogens (even those for which an experimental NOEL for other toxic effects has been determined), the dose-response data are treated differently. The size of the increase in toxic effects at various low doses, where the risk per animal (and by extension, per person exposed) is quite small, is generally of greatest interest but not directly observable because of practical limits on experimentation. Carcinogenicity data from animal studies generally show that increasingly high doses cause a corresponding increase in the incidence of cancers. However, the doses used in animals are exceedingly high in terms of human risk to compensate for the fact that only small numbers of animals can be used in experimentation of this type (OSTP, 1985). For example, if 50 animals are exposed to a dose of a carcinogen and 5 develop tumors, the risk is 10% (if no control animals develop a tumor). A cancer risk near 10% would be intolerable in any human setting, but this is about the smallest risk that can be reliably detected in animal experiments of practicable size (OSTP, 1985).

The experimentally determined relationship between dose and risk at high doses must therefore be used to assess risk for dose levels corresponding to human exposures. This requires the use of certain mathematical models of the dose-response data (FSC, 1980; NRC, 1980b; OSTP, 1985). These models generally provide unit risk estimates, i.e., estimates of cancer risk per unit of dose (such as the incidence of cancer at a dose of 1 mg/kg bw/day over a lifetime). The models most widely used for low dose carcinogenic risk assessment are based on assumptions that there is no threshold and that risk at very low doses increases in direct proportion to dose. Several models meet this criterion. EPA uses the linearized multistage model, which incorporates an upper 95% confidence limit on the estimated linear term. Table 5-1 presents risks per unit of low dose exposure predicted by this model for substances that are potential contaminants of poultry products. Models used by FDA and the National Research Council's Safe Drinking Water Committee (NRC, 1980a) would yield unit cancer risks close to those shown in Table 5-1.

It is not possible to demonstrate that any mathematical models are fully in accord with biological reality. Because this subject has been discussed elsewhere (NRC, 1980a; OSTP, 1985), the committee simply notes in this report that certain models are widely used in risk prediction and that they are generally interpreted on the basis of little direct evidence as providing upper limits on low dose risk, although recent data suggest that this may sometimes be wrong (J. C. Bailar, Harvard School of Public Health, personal communication, 1987). Policy choices needed in the face of scientific uncertainty have also been discussed in another National Research Council report (NRC, 1980b).

The dose-response assessment phase of risk assessment thus generally concludes with a determination of NOELs (for noncarcinogenic effects) and of estimates of risk per unit dose (unit risks) for cancers. In both determinations there are important uncertainties that need to be specified in the report of the risk assessment. Since many of these uncertainties concern the data on which these dose-response estimates are based and are therefore chemical-specific, they must be defined by experts who have studied a specific substance. Other uncertainties are generic (e.g., some are inherent in models for extrapolating from high to low doses) and therefore apply to all chemicals.

Exposure Assessment

Exposure assessment is a highly complex subject, and is reviewed here only to the extent necessary to prepare for the later discussion of chemical residues in poultry products. In this phase of risk assessment, knowledge of the magnitude and duration of human exposure to environmental agents and, most importantly, the dose that results from this exposure, is essential. As used herein, the term exposure describes a person's contact with a medium (e.g., poultry) containing a chemical. The magnitude of the dose that results from the exposure depends on several factors, which are described in the following paragraphs.

To estimate dose, the possible routes of chemical intake must first be identified. For residues in poultry, ingestion is the only route of concern. Occupational exposures might include inhalation, dermal contact, or other routes of exposure, but these routes are not germane

TABLE 5-1 Unit Cancer Risks and Strength-of-Evidence Categories for 47 Chemicals, as Evaluated by the EPA Carcinogen Assessment' Group[a]

Compound	Level of Evidence[b]		Unit Cancer Risk per mg/kg bw/day[c]
	Humans	Animals	
Acrylonitrile	L	S	0.24(W)
Aflatoxin B$_1$	L	S	2,900
Aldrin	I	L	11.4
Allyl chloride	—	—	1.19×10^{-2}
Arsenic	S	I	15(H)
Benzo[a]pyrene	I	S	11.5
Benzene	S	S	2.9×10^{-2}(W)
Benzidene	S	S	234(W)
Beryllium	L	S	2.6(W)
Cadmium	L	S	6.1(W)
Carbon tetrachloride	I	S	1.30×10^{-1}
Chlordane	I	L	1.61
Chlorinated ethanes:			
1,2-Dichloroethane	I	S	9.1×10^{-2}
Hexachloroethane	I	L	1.42×10^{-2}
1,1,2,2-Tetrachloroethane	I	L	0.20
1,1,2-Trichloroethane	I	L	5.73×10^{-2}
Chloroform	I	S	8.1×10^{-2}
Chromium VI	S	S	41(W)
Dichlorodiphenyltrichloroethane (DDT)	I	S	0.34
Dichlorobenzidine	I	S	1.69

	Level of Evidence[b]		
Compound	Humans	Animals	Unit Cancer Risk per mg/kg bw/day[c]
Dieldrin	I	S	30.4
Epichlorohydrin	I	S	9.9×10^{-3}
Bis(2-chloroethyl)ether	I	S	1.14
Bis(chloromethyl)ether	S	S	9,300(In)
Ethylene dibromide	I	S	41
Ethylene oxide	L	S	3.5×10^{-1}(In)
Heptachlor	I	S	3.37
Hexachlorobenzene	I	S	1.67
Hexachlorobutadiene	I	L	7.75×10^{-2}
Hexachlorocyclohexane:			
Technical grade	—	—	4.75
Alpha isomer	I	S	11.12
Beta isomer	I	L	1.84
Gamma isomer	I	L	1.33
Nickel refinery dust	S	S	1.05(W)
Nitrosamines:			
Dimethylnitrosamine	I	S	25.9(not by q*)[d]
Diethylnitrosamine	I	S	43 5(not by q*)
Dibutylnitrosamine	I	S	5.43
N-Nitrosopyrrolidine	I	S	2.13
N-Nitroso-N-ethylurea	I	S	32.9
N-Nitroso-N-methylurea	I	S	302.6
Polychlorinated biphenyls (PCBs)	I	S	4.34
Phenols:			
2,4,6-Trichlorophenol	I	S	1.99×10^{-2}
Tetrachlorodibenzo-p-dioxin (TCCD)	I	S	$1.56 \times 10^{+5}$

	Level of Evidence[b]		
Coumpound	Humans	Animals	Unit Cancer Rick per mg/kg bw/day[c]
Tetrachloroethylene	I	L	5.1×10^{-2}
Toxaphene	I	S	1.13
Trichloroethylene	I	L/S	1.1×10^{-2}
Vinyl chloride	S	S	1.75×10^{-2} (In)

[a] Adapted from EPA, 1985.

[b] S = Sufficient evidence; L = Limited evidence; I = Inadequate evidence, according to the International Agency for Research on Cancer.

[c] UCRs are 95% upper-limit slopes based on the linearized multistage model. Calculations of these slopes are based on data from oral studies in animals except for those indicated by In (animal inhalation), W (human occupational exposure), and H (human drinking water exposure). Slopes for humans are point estimates based on the linear nonthreshold model. Not all of the carcinogenic potencies presented in this table represent the same degree of certainty. All are subject to change as new evidence becomes available.

[d] q* is the 95% upper-bound confidence limit of the linear parameter.

in this report. Exposure assessment is designed to yield dose estimates for both short-term and long-term studies.

Daily doses of chemical residues received by humans through poultry consumption are estimated by determining the chemical concentrations in various poultry products and the average daily intake of each product. FSIS's National Residue Monitoring Program has collected information on 20 chemicals found as residues in young chicken carcass samples examined from 1979 to 1984 (Table 5-2).

Internal absorption also influences dose. Ingested substances must pass through the gastrointestinal wall to produce systemic effects, but there are differences in the rate and completeness with which different substances pass through this barrier. Direct measurements of absorption are rarely available and cannot be obtained without conducting experimental studies in humans. Therefore, it is common either to adopt absorption rates from animal studies of compounds with similar chemical and physical characteristics or to assume that absorption is complete (Calabrese, 1983; Nisbet, 1981).

Precise identification of the population to which the risk assessment will be applied is another important requirement of exposure assessment. This may be the general population or a special subpopulation, such as infants, believed to be at special risk. In this chapter it is assumed that the general population will be exposed to chemical residues in poultry, but the concept and principles described herein apply just as well to any defined subpopulation.

The general population contains not only healthy adults but also infants, children, pregnant women, the elderly, the immunosuppressed, and the chronically ill, which represent the full range of susceptibilities to a toxic agent. In such a population, there is likely to be a wider range of responses to a toxic agent than in a group consisting primarily of healthy adult males, e.g., certain worker groups. Risk assessment based on animal data from highly controlled experiments (e.g., studies using inbred strains, homogenized feed, or uniform holding conditions, or excluding other agents that might act synergistically with the test substances) will reflect an even narrower range of susceptibilities. For risk assessment, therefore, it is important to know the characteristics of the exposed population. Finally, for toxic agents with thresholds and for most nonthreshold carcinogens it is important to know not only the mean dose received by the population but also the distribution of doses, if one is to determine whether even the most highly exposed individuals are exposed to subthreshold doses.

Risk Characterization

Noncarcinogens. Since there are no methods for estimating risks for low doses of noncarcinogens, it has become the practice to divide the experimentally determined NOEL for these substances by a large

Table 5-2. Examples of Chemical Residues in Young Chickens[a]

Chemical and Year Reported	Tissue	Number of Contaminated Samples Found, by Concentration (ppm)								
		0	0.01-0.10	0.11-0.20	0.21-0.30	0.31-0.50	0.51-1.00	1.01-2.00	2.01-2.50	2.51-5.00
PESTICIDES:										
Benzene-hexachloride:										
1981	Fat	467	5							
1982	Fat	432	2							
1983	Fat	422	2							
1984	Fat	448	6							
Chlordane:										
1981	Fat	469	3							
1982	Fat	433	1							
1983	Fat	420	3			1				
Dieldrin:										
1979	Fat	221	10	1						
1980	Fat	582		14[b]						
1981	Fat	458	14							
1982	Fat	426	7							
1983	Fat	412	12							
1984	Fat	428	26							
DDT:										
1979	Fat	211	19	1	1					
1980	Fat	502		92[b]			2[c]			
1981	Fat	409	60	2	1					
1982	Fat	414	19	1						
1983	Fat	375	45	2			2			
1984	Fat	391	61	1					1	
Endrin:										
1980	Fat	595		1[b]						
1981	Fat	470	2							
1984	Fat	452	2							
Heptachlor:										
1979	Fat	231	1							
1980	Fat	590		6[b]						
1981	Fat	768	4							
1983	Fat	422	1	1						
1984	Fat	447	7							
Lindane:										
1979	Fat	231	1							
1980	Fat	588		8[b]						
1981	Fat	470	2	1						
1983	Fat	421	2	1						
1984	Fat	447	7							
Methoxychlor:										
1979	Fat	231	1							
1984	Fat	452		1				1		
Polychlorinated biphenyls:										
1983	Fat	423				1				

[a]From FSIS, National Residue Monitoring Program, unpublished data, 1979-1984.
[b]A concentration range of 0.01-0.30 ppm was reported.

Chemical and Year Reported	Tissue	0	0.01-0.10	0.11-0.20	0.21-0.30	0 31-0.50	0.51-1.00	1.01-2.00	2.01-2.50	2.51-5.00
PESTICIDES (cont.)										
Hydroxychlorinated biphenyls:										
1979	Fat	225	7							
1980	Fat	588		8[b]						
1981	Fat	469	3							
1984	Fat	450	4							
p-Chlorophenol:										
1981	Liver	0	6	3						
1983	Liver	247					9	1	1	1
ENVIRONMENTAL CONTAMINANTS:										
Arsenic:										
1979	Liver	42	15	15	23	46	81	30		
1980	Liver	41		51[b]		230[c]	43[d]	3[e]	4	
1981	Liver	30	23	17	42	103	152	39	2	1
1982	Liver	30	14	10	22	71	82	16	1	
1984	Liver	50	11	12	19	77	130	28		
1979	Muscle	1	1	1						
1980	Muscle	0		6[b]		1[c]				
1981	Muscle	41	48	4	1					
1982	Muscle		1				1			
1984	Muscle		1				1			
Mercury:										
1979	Liver								1	
Selenium:										
1979	Liver					4	7	1		
1979	Muscle		4	3	3	1	1			
1979	Kidney					1	6	5		
PHARMACEUTICALS AND ANTIBIOTICS:										
Chlortetracycline:										
1984	Liver	3	1							
1982	Kidney	393	1							
1984	Kidney	274	2							
Decoquinate:										
1983	Liver	198								
Oxytetracycline:										
1983	Kidney	342								
Pyrantel tartrate:										
1983	Liver	38	24	11	17	72	169	63		
1983	Muscle	2		2						
Sulfadimethoxine:										
1981	Kidney	313				1				
1982	Kidney	286	1							
Sulfquimoxaline:										
1981	Liver	4		1						
1981	Kidney	312		1	1					
1982	Kidney	286	1							

[c] A concentration range of 0.31-1.00 ppm was reported.
[d] A concentration range of 1.01-1.50 ppm was reported.
[e] A concentration range of 1.51-2.00 ppm was reported.

safety factor to estimate acceptable human doses (i.e., acceptable daily intake, or ADI). This method was first used during the 1940s and 1950s to regulate food additives and pesticides (Lehman and Fitzhugh, 1954) and has since been extended to other categories, such as drinking water contaminants (NRC 1977, 1980a).

The safety factor approach is based on several considerations. One is statistical; that is, a small sample of animals is not likely to exhibit a statistically significant number of reactions at some low dose even if the frequency with which such reactions occur is high enough to be of major concern in the human population. Another consideration is the likelihood that a human population will have a wider range of susceptibilities than the test animal group from which the NOEL is obtained. The human population is genetically more diverse than study groups of laboratory animals and contains certain subgroups (e.g., infants and the ill) that are likely to be more susceptible than healthy test animals. The human population is also exposed to a wider range of other environmental agents and lifestyle factors, e.g., it includes people who smoke, drink alcoholic beverages, and take medicines. Because of such additional exposures, the background of risk for human populations is different and often higher than that of test animals and may generally increase the susceptibility of the human population in comparison to test animals. It is also likely that the variation in threshold doses (doses below which no toxic response is observed) for a particular substance will vary more widely in the human population than in a small, genetically and experimentally homogeneous animal group.

For these reasons, the threshold dose for the human population is likely to be lower than that approximated by the NOEL derived from studies in animals. To take into account all the uncertainties about the relative susceptibilities of the human and animal populations as well as the wide range of susceptibilities within the human population, the experimental NOEL is divided by a safety factor to derive an ADI for humans. If the NOEL is based on the results of a well-conducted chronic toxicity study and relates to an effect other than cancer, a safety factor of 100 is usually applied (NRC, 1980a). If NOELs have been estimated for several animal species, the value for the most sensitive species (i.e., the lowest value of NOEL) is used to estimate the safe level for humans. For example, if a substance has been shown in chronic studies to cause liver damage in rats at high doses, and if the experimental NOEL for this effect is 100 mg/kg bw/day, the ADI is set at 1 mg/kg bw/day. This ADI is considered safe for humans in the sense that there is little likelihood of a toxic response in members of the human population exposed daily to the 1 mg/kg dose (NRC, 1980a). If humans are exposed to an agent having this ADI, and if it is assumed, for example, that their exposure comes solely through ingestion of drinking water, that their weight is 60 kg, and that they drink 2 liters of water per day, then a 30 mg/liter concentration of this agent in drinking water would be considered acceptably safe.[1]

---

[1] Calculated as follows: 30 mg/liter × 2 liters/day = 60 mg intake per day. 60 mg/day ÷ 60 kg bw = 1 mg/kg bw/day.

A more refined calculation is needed if one is to consider additional sources of exposure. For example, if intake of a substance with an ADI of 1 mg/kg bw derives from both ingestion of 2 liters of water per day and consumption of contaminated poultry products, then 30 mg/liter in water would not be considered safe. To decide what level of contaminants could be permitted in both water and poultry so that the ADI would not be exceeded, it is necessary to know the daily intake of both water and poultry products and to make a policy decision about how to apportion the ADI between these two sources.

Safety factors larger than 100 are commonly used when data on humans are not available and experimental data are limited (Calabrese, 1983; EPA, 1980; FDA, 1982b; NRC, 1986). For example, a factor of 1,000 is used for NOELs derived from subchronic toxicity studies when no chronic data are available (NRC, 1980b). Larger factors may also be used for especially serious effects, such as cancer or birth defects. Teratogens may be effective following just a few exposures during critical times during pregnancy. Teratogenicity might be regarded as a form of acute toxicity, but the effects are permanent. Smaller safety factors are sometimes used for certain populations (e.g., relatively healthy, adult worker populations) believed to be less vulnerable than the general population and, rarely, when adequate data on NOELs are available from studies in human populations.

In a distinct but related approach, risk characterization for noncarcinogens is accomplished by determining the margin of safety (MOS), that is, the numerical value derived when the experimental NOEL is divided by the actual human dose. A judgment is then needed to determine whether the MOS is sufficiently large to protect most members of the exposed population. Guidance on the adequacy of a given MOS can be obtained by comparing the commonly used safety factors for establishing ADIs to the MOS. For chronic toxicity, an MOS of 100 might be considered adequate, assuming that the data are adequate. There is an element of policy in the selection of safety margins, and any standard-setting activity should be seen to have a risk-management component.

Under this system, the smaller the value of the MOS, the larger the risk. If the MOS is close to one, many members of the exposed population might be at high risk of toxicity. This is not true when the effects and dose-response characteristics of a substance are well-established in humans. Some air pollutants (e.g., carbon monoxide) can be protected against by using relatively small MOSs. If the MOS is only a small fraction of the NOEL, the risk may be low or zero, but there is no way to determine with complete certainty whether this is the case. Conversely, occasional exposures exceeding the ADI may not be associated with any risk at all. The limitations and uncertainties of this system are discussed later in this chapter.

Carcinogens. If a unit cancer risk (UCR), i.e., risk per unit dose, has been determined for a carcinogen, this value is multiplied by the average daily lifetime human dose to derive an estimate of risk. In this case, the risk is estimated, and its value ranges from 0 and 1. Even for well-studied carcinogens, this estimate of risk is uncertain and it can not be claimed to be the true risk. EPA and FDA state that these values are upper bound risks and that the true risk is likely to be less. Despite the uncertainties, numerical estimates of risk are commonly used as decision-making tools for separating significant from negligible risks (NRC, 1980b; Rodricks and Taylor, 1983).

USES OF RISK ASSESSMENT IN STANDARD SETTING

Some standards are based on assessments performed by the methods described above. Following are some examples of the use of risk assessment in the setting of standards, some of which can apply to poultry products.

Food and Color Additives

FDA establishes ADIs based on data submitted by industry and application of the methods described above. Under law, no ADI can be established for carcinogens directly added to food including poultry (thus, no carcinogen can be directly added to food). For certain classes of unavoidable food constituents that are carcinogenic, FDA has permitted residue levels corresponding to doses presenting a negligible lifetime cancer risk as estimated by the methods described above (FDA, 1982a). FDA not only requires that the total human dose from all uses of an additive not exceed the ADI, but also that limits (tolerances) for additives be set at the lowest level at which the desired technical effect will be produced.

Animal Drug Residues on Food

FDA establishes ADIs for animal drug residues using the procedures described above for food and color additives. Tolerances for residues in individual tissues are based on the expected distribution and concentrations of residues in poultry products (learned from metabolism and pharmacokinetic studies) and on the criterion that all sources of exposure together do not exceed the ADI. Carcinogenic drug residues are permitted up to a level corresponding to an upper limit lifetime risk of 1 in a million (FDA, 1985).

Pesticide Residues on Food

EPA uses the same risk-assessment methodology used by FDA for food and color additives and applies it to data submitted by industry. An upper-bound lifetime risk of 1 in a million is used as a guide for determining acceptable residue levels of carcinogenic pesticides that do not meet the legal definition of a food additive, and risk-benefit balancing is a part of EPA's standard-setting procedure. ADIs are used for noncarcinogens.

Environmental Contaminants

Food and other media may be contaminated with certain organic and inorganic chemicals of both industrial and natural origin. Limits on such agents in food, including meat and poultry products, are established by FDA. ADIs may be established, but standard safety factors may not always be used. This is especially true for various metals that present a substantial background exposure. For carcinogens, risks higher than those accepted for additives have sometimes been tolerated (see, e.g., FDA limits on PCBs in fish; FDA, 1979). Tolerances for poultry products should take into account the magnitude of all other exposures to the same and related substances. Industry has not had to supply all the data necessary to establish acceptable limits on exposure, although some relevant data are submitted to EPA or required by the Toxic Substances Control Act.

LIMITATIONS AND UNCERTAINTIES IN RISK ASSESSMENT

Assessments of risks are based on data that vary in quality and quantity among different environmental chemicals. Some chemicals have been tested for toxicity far more extensively than others, often because of regulatory requirements for such testing in certain classes of chemicals before they can be accepted into commerce (e.g., pesticides, food and color additives, drugs).

The Toxic Substances Control Act stipulates similar testing requirements for other classes of chemicals in commerce, primarily chemicals newly proposed for substantial commercial applications. The Department of Health and Human Services's National Toxicology Program is also producing data on commercial products but is limited largely to carcinogenicity testing. Despite these testing programs, it will probably be many years before a relatively complete and uniform toxicity data base will be available for these commercially important substances (NRC, 1984).

The inadequacies in both quality and quantity of data for many different chemicals introduce uncertainty, and the type and degree of uncertainty vary from one substance to another. For example, one chemical may have been well tested for subchronic toxicity but its possible carcinogenic effects may not have been studied, whereas another substance may have been tested for carcinogenicity but not for teratogenic effects.

Test quality is another important consideration. Exposures of many people to high levels of a substance that appears not to be carcinogenic but has not been fully tested in adequately designed animal studies may be of greater concern than low levels of exposures of a few people to a substance found to be weakly carcinogenic in a well-designed study in animals. There are no hard-and-fast rules to guide assessment of such exposures. As a result, many of the uncertainties in risk assessment are chemical-specific (e.g., data on the magnitude of human exposure) and cannot be reduced to general statements. An adequate risk assessment should contain a description of all the uncertainties and how they were considered in arriving at conclusions about risk.

Risk assessments are also based on certain biologically plausible, as yet untested assumptions and inferences. Among the more important inferences are those concerning similarities between humans and test animals and the nature of dose-response functions at dose levels well below the observable range of experimental dose-response relationships (see above section on Dose-Response Assessment).

In the absence of information about toxicity in humans, it is biologically plausible to divide NOELs for animals by certain safety factors (see above section on Risk Characterization), but there is little empirical information for use in determining the most appropriate factor. In fact, without quantitative data on dose-response relationships for specific substances in humans, it is not possible to determine the quantitative difference in toxic response, if any, between human populations and test animal groups. Safety factors have come to be used to compensate for these gaps in fundamental knowledge.

The methods of risk assessment discussed above are widely used by regulatory agencies and committees of NRC. Although these methods cannot remove scientific uncertainty, they ensure that the risk assessments properly reflect the best available scientific knowledge. There are no known superior methods for assessing the risk to public health.

Application of these methods and determination of acceptable risks for carcinogens or acceptable intakes for other substances based on decisions about acceptable MOSs are designed to ensure that no significant risk is imposed on populations. In most cases, this goal is untested (and may be largely untestable because of the extreme difficulty in acquiring quantitative toxicity data in humans). Nonetheless, it serves as the basis of various health protection standards.

CHEMICAL RESIDUES IN POULTRY PRODUCTS AND THEIR PUBLIC HEALTH RISKS

Sources and Types

The 1985 NRC report on meat and poultry inspection included a survey of the various types of chemicals that are used in meat and poultry production or that may occur as inadvertent contaminants (NRC, 1985). For present purposes it is not necessary to duplicate that survey, but only to organize the information in a form more convenient for application to poultry products and to develop a strategy for risk assessment. A useful approach is to examine the various ways in which chemicals come to be present in poultry products. These can be divided into four major classes:

Class 1. Legally approved (e.g., by FDA or USDA) chemicals intentionally administered or applied to poultry or to feeds used for poultry. These include, for example, the pesticides, pharmaceuticals, and antibiotics listed in Table 5-2 as well as chemicals used in processing, such as sodium benzoate, potassium sorbate, and monosodium glutamate; feed additives, such as butylated hydroxyanisole, butylated hydroxytoluene, nitrates, and nitrites; and certain growth promoters.

Class 2. Widespread environmental contaminants to which poultry may be exposed because of their presence in poultry feed or drinking water. These include organic and inorganic chemicals of industrial or natural origin, including pesticides that are present in media for which there is no registered use. Among the possible organic contaminants are polychlorinated biphenyls, polychlorinated dioxins and benzofurans, chlordane, dieldrin, heptachlor, dichlorodiphenyl-trichloroethane, and lindane. Among the inorganic compounds are mercury and arsenic. Mycotoxins such as aflatoxins are also included in this class.

Class 3. Chemicals to which poultry may be exposed as a result of accidental contamination. These may be any of the chemicals in Classes 1 and 2 and many other substances in commercial production.

Class 4. Chemicals formed when poultry is processed (chlorine, polyvinyl chloride, acrylonitrile), stored (fatty acid hydroperoxides, hydroperoxyl radicals), and cooked at high temperatures (amino-carboline congeners, polycyclic aromatic hydrocarbons).

This classification is especially useful both for risk assessment and risk management. Perhaps different risk-management strategies should be used for each of the four classes, which are distinguishable in the following ways:

- All substances in Class 1 can legally be used only in compliance with preestablished regulations based on the types of risk assessment and standard-setting procedures described above. There may or may not be such regulations for substances in Classes 2, 3, or 4.
- The degree to which residues of the four classes can be predicted to occur in poultry varies greatly. Generally, Class 1 substances are highly predictable, Class 3 substances are highly unpredictable, and Class 2 and 4 substances fall between these extremes.
- Class 1 substances should not be expected to present high risks unless the preestablished tolerances or limits are repeatedly

violated because of intentional or accidental misuse. The risks of Class 2, 3, and 4 substances without preestablished exposure limits cannot be readily judged without a great deal more information than currently exists about their toxic properties and their occurrence in poultry products and other environmental media.

- For substances in Classes 1, 2, and 4, the principal concern is the risk of chronic exposure. The risk of acute exposure is the major concern for Class 3 substances.
- The quality and completeness of the toxicological data base used to establish acceptable intake levels are likely to be good for Class 1 substances and generally inadequate for all but a few substances in Classes 2, 3, and 4.
- Knowledge of the number and identities of chemicals in Class 1 is very good. It is significantly less complete for Class 2 chemicals and highly imperfect for Class 3 and 4 substances.
- The availability of reliable, sensitive, and practical analytical methods for measuring the chemicals in the four classes varies greatly. Methods for Class 1 chemicals are probably superior to those in the other classes. For many substances in Classes 2, 3, and 4, there are no methods available.

Each of these factors plays a role in risk assessment and risk management.

Type and Magnitude of Risk

For some purposes, it is useful to organize chemicals according to type and magnitude of risk, rather than by source, especially when one must estimate overall public health risk from chemical residues from all sources. To accomplish this, it would be necessary to identify the toxic properties of chemicals known to occupy one or more of the four classes and to regroup them according to their types of toxicity. Traditional categories of toxicants, such as carcinogens, teratogens, liver toxicants, kidney toxicants, and reproductive toxicants, could be used for this purpose. The methods of risk assessment described above could then be applied to residue concentration data and information on human intake of poultry products to estimate the public health risk posed by chemical residues in poultry products. This approach is discussed further in the last section of this chapter.

Although categorization of risk by type and magnitude is an important component of a risk-assessment program for poultry, there are important reasons to use source of residue classification as the principal system, which serves as the basis of the following discussion.

USING RISK ASSESSMENT TO ESTABLISH RISK-MANAGEMENT PROGRAMS

Risk assessments are generally undertaken as a basis for risk management, i.e., the process of controlling risks so they are at acceptable levels. This is especially true for FSIS's assessment of risks presented by chemical residues in poultry. Effective prevention of such risks to public health requires the following types of activities:

1. Identifying substances that could appear as residues in poultry.
2. Setting ADIs or other levels of tolerable daily intake using the tools of risk assessment.
3. Establishing tolerances for residue levels in edible poultry products, taking into account other sources of human exposure so that the ADI (or tolerable intake level) is not exceeded.
4. Setting levels of chemical intake by poultry (through their diets, drinking water, or other sources) that will ensure that tolerance levels in poultry products are not exceeded.
5. Establishing quality control programs to ensure that poultry feeds, drinking water, or other sources do not contain the chemicals of concern at levels exceeding those identified in Activity 4.
6. Establishing monitoring programs to ensure that poultry products reaching consumers do not contain residues above the limits established in Activity 3.
7. Establishing enforcement procedures to provide efficient deterrence and, when needed, to ensure removal of contaminated poultry products from commerce.
8. Identifying priorities for the different steps in each of these activities by using the concepts and tools of risk assessment.

Given the present state of knowledge, these tasks cannot be accomplished for all classes of residues with equal rigor and certainty. However, it is important to begin them to assess the extent to which each is currently being undertaken and to manage known potential risks in the most efficent way.

The risks of Class 4 substances are poorly understood, and the efforts needed to identify and deal with them are substantially different from those needed for the other classes. Thus, chemicals in that class, i.e., those formed during processing, storing, and heating, are omitted from this discussion and are included in a separate section on Special Problems later in the chapter.

In the following discussion of the eight activities described above, no attempt is made to identify responsibility unless it is clear that such responsibility already exists (e.g., EPA's responsibility to assign tolerances for pesticide residues). The options for carrying out the various risk assessment and management tasks are discussed in later chapters of this report.

Activity 1. Identifying Chemicals of Potential Concern

<u>Class 1 Chemicals</u>. The use of such substances is based on information about their toxic properties and the levels of residues expected to occur in poultry products as well as demonstration to the satisfaction of EPA, FDA, or FSIS that no significant risk will result under specific conditions of use. This information, including approved use conditions, is specified in formal regulations (for a typical example, see CFR, 1986, which concerns the use of a sulfonamide drug in swine). There is no reason to believe that any chemicals in this class have escaped identification. Class 1 chemicals introduced in the future are expected to be similarly well identified.

Unidentified metabolites or degradation products of Class 1 chemicals may occur as residues, however, and are not taken into account in established tolerances. This potential applies to all classes and is discussed later in this chapter along with Class 4 substances under Special Problems.

<u>Class 2 Chemicals</u>. EPA has collected information on many potential inorganic and organic contaminants of drinking water and has established maximum contaminant levels for many but not all of them. EPA, FDA, and USDA have collected information on some of the known contaminants of feed ingredients, and FSIS has gathered some data on residues in poultry products.

It will be necessary to conduct an extensive literature review to identify regular contaminants of drinking water used in the production and processing of poultry and contaminants of all ingredients used in poultry feed. In this way it should be possible to ensure that all important chemicals in Class 2 have been identified.

Some Class 2 substances can reasonably be treated as chemical classes. Polychlorinated biphenyls (PCBs), for example, are mixtures of closely related substances that share toxic properties. PCBs have been subjected to toxicity testing as mixtures, and data from these tests have been used to estimate the risks presented by these mixtures. For other chemicals (e.g., chlorinated ethanes), there are data on individual, closely related chemicals. If these chemicals produce similar forms of toxicity, they may be treated as a class for risk assessment.

As part of this activity, it is necessary to gather any data that bear on the toxicological properties of these chemicals in poultry. Of particular concern are data suggesting that any of these contaminants can accumulate in edible animal tissues. Information on bioaccumulation need not be obtained only from studies in poultry, but can be derived from studies in other animal species as well.

All this information can be used to produce an initial list of chemicals in Class 2, which can be updated as new data emerge, and to develop a scale of the relative probabilities that those chemicals may occur as residues in poultry products. These relative probabilities can be used to set priorities for the remaining risk-assessment and management activities.

A surveillance program will be needed to determine the actual occurrence of these residues in poultry products. This program should include poultry sampling and analysis to identify problems. It should not be used to monitor for compliance with established limits.

Class 3 Chemicals. A systematic attempt should be made to identify substances that lead to product contamination through occasional misuse or accidents. Information useful in identifying such chemicals include historical and current reports on accidental exposure of poultry and accidental contamination of poultry products, drinking water, and poultry feed ingredients. Also useful are data on industrial activities in the vicinity of poultry production facilities and feed production operations.

This type of information, which is available from several sources (e.g., EPA, FDA, USDA, various state agencies, and the scientific literature), can be used to determine whether specific groups of chemicals, including those in Class 1, are especially likely to be accidentally released in ways that may lead to contamination of water and feed ingredients.

Activity 2. Risk Assessment to Identify ADIs or Other Tolerable Intake Levels

Class 1 Chemicals. Risk assessments have been carried out on most if not all substances in this class—by FDA for feed additives and drug residues in poultry and by EPA for pesticide residues—with methods similar to those described above. Use of substances in this class under conditions prescribed in regulations should not lead to residue levels that exceed tolerances. This should in turn ensure that ADIs or other tolerable intake levels are not exceeded.

The degree to which the toxicological data on chemicals in Class 1 meet currently accepted standards of quality and completeness is unknown to this committee, and can not be determined without a thorough review of data in FDA and EPA files. Information reviewed in the NRC report on meat and poultry inspection suggests that there are substantial inadequacies in the data base (NRC, 1985). Thus, the data on Class 1 substances should be continually reviewed to determine whether current standards have been adequately satisfied. Only then can FSIS or any other agency determine with confidence whether compliance with current exposure limits ensures adequate public health protection.

The committee reviewed the data and found no evidence to suggest either that current exposure limits for Class 1 substances fail to protect the public health or that the poultry industry does not attempt to comply with these limits. In the absence of firm information about the adequacy of the data bases, however, the committee cannot conclude unequivocally that compliance with current limits is adequate to protect public health.

Class 2 Substances. Extensive data on toxicity are available for some potential members of Class 2 (e.g., certain metals, PCBs, dioxins, aflatoxins), and the data bases have been thoroughly evaluated by groups such as EPA, FDA, WHO, and NRC. For other substances that might be in Class 2, the toxicological data base is quite inadequate. More specific statements about the adequacy of the data cannot be made without a thorough literature review, which should make it possible to separate substances for which adequate risk assessments can be performed from those requiring additional toxicological data.

Because substances in Class 2 are widespread environmental contaminants, chronic human exposure is possible. It is therefore important to ensure the adequacy of the toxicological data base for estimating limits on chronic exposure. Once the necessary data are available, risk assessments can be performed for this class as they are for Class 1 substances. Because environmental exposure to some Class 2 chemicals is widespread, the degree of acceptable risk may be higher for some Class 1 substances (e.g., noncarcinogens) than for others (e.g., carcinogens). EPA, FDA, and WHO have considered this when setting acceptable levels for PCBs in fish, for metals in certain foods and drinking water, and for aflatoxins in peanut and corn products. The types of risk-management analysis necessary to decide when to depart from the limits usually imposed on Class 1 substances are beyond the scope of the present study but need to be recognized.

Class 3 Chemicals. In contrast to Classes 1 and 2, a major concern for Class 3 substances is short-term, occasional exposures, e.g., those that might result from a chemical spill. Short-term dietary exposure limits should be established for substances, including those in Classes 1 and 2, with a high probability of misuse or accidental contamination of diet. Methods for estimating short-term limits are similar to those for estimating ADIs, except that the data requirements are substantially reduced. Methods for establishing such limits have been reviewed by NRC committees (NRC, 1983).

Activity 3. Estimating Tolerances in Edible Poultry Products

For each substance for which an ADI, short-term exposure limit, or other exposure limit is established, it is necessary to identify the maximum concentration, or tolerances, to be allowed in edible poultry products. To establish such tolerances, it is necessary to know the amount of each poultry product (typically muscle, skin, liver, and kidney) consumed each day by members of the population and other sources of human exposure to the same chemical or class of chemicals (diet and drinking water but possibly through air and soil as well).

Data on poultry consumption rates have been estimated for different segments of the population, e.g., the average consumer and the 90th percentile consumer. The segment used to define tolerances should be objectively selected and explicitly defined; some precedents for the selection process have already been established by FDA and EPA. Any differences among agencies in consumption data and their uses should be identified and resolved.

For substances in Class 1, data on other exposures are usually taken into account by FDA and EPA when tolerances are set, but it is not clear to the committee whether this has been done adequately, for example, whether data on groundwater contamination by pesticides were adequately considered in setting tolerances for the same pesticides in edible animal products. All information on human exposure to Class 1 and 2 substances should be used in setting the maximum tolerable daily intake or ADI for poultry products. The portion of allowable total exposure that should be allocated to poultry products and other media should be determined jointly by all concerned regulatory agencies.

The concern is to set tolerances for relatively high exposures of short duration. Since the chronic background exposure level is ordinarily comparatively insignificant, it is not generally necessary to consider other exposure sources.

Activity 4. Identifying Acceptable Levels of Chemical Intake for Poultry

It is desirable to identify the maximum level of daily chemical intake (through feed or drinking water) that can be tolerated by poultry to ensure that residue levels do not exceed tolerances. With such information, it would be possible to monitor poultry feed and drinking water as an alternative to, or in addition to, monitoring poultry products. Among other benefits, complete information on the association between intake of chemicals and residue levels in poultry products would probably reduce the need for using safety factors in the assessment of risks for feed and water. However, a risk-management program can operate without this information and, indeed, should not fail to operate if the information is not available.

Acceptable exposure levels may of course change over time as a flock matures. The acceptable intake may be set at zero for some period before slaughter (withdrawal period).

Class 1 Chemicals. FDA and EPA generally require that metabolic and pharmacokinetic studies be conducted to establish exposure limits for substances in Class 1. These studies are designed to identify the levels in feed or water or levels of drug administration. The data from these studies can then be used to establish tolerance levels for Class 1 substances in drinking water or feed. The adequacy of the toxicological data base for establishing feed or drinking water tolerances for Class 1 substances is discussed under Activity 2.

Class 2 Chemicals. Control of feed and water contamination may be the most effective strategy for managing the risks presented by Class 2 substances, but only a few of the common substances in this class, e.g., aflatoxin, PCBs, and certain heavy metals, have been carefully studied to measure the relationship between feed or drinking water levels and levels in edible poultry products. One reason for this is that poultry cannot be held in storage during the slow process of chemical analysis. It is especially important that this information be collected and analyzed immediately. However, without the necessary metabolic and pharmacokinetic data, suitable feed and water tolerances cannot be established. For only a few substances, there are sufficient data for estimating the maximum chemical concentrations in feed, water, or both that will not lead to violation of tolerances in poultry products. Both feed and water tolerances may be necessary for some Class 2 substances (e.g., metals), because both media may be pathways of poultry exposure.

Class 3 Chemicals. The data needed for Class 3 substances can be acquired through study of the biological disposition and excretion rates of chemicals in poultry following short-term, high-level exposures. Such data can be used to identify potentially dangerous levels in feed or water.

Activity 5. Feed and Water Quality Control

A risk-management program based on tolerances in poultry feed and water, coupled with quality control and enforcement that is adequate to ensure that the tolerances are met, might be substantially more effective than a program based on monitoring of residues in poultry products. As long as feed and water tolerances are met, one could reasonably assume that residue levels in poultry products do not exceed established tolerances. This program would correct problems before they occur and seems to be especially well suited to the well-controlled conditions under which most poultry are now raised. If such a program were in effect, however, monitoring of poultry products would still be necessary but would not constitute the principal risk-management tool.

Routine monitoring for Class 1 and 2 chemical contamination of feed and water could be required. Priorities for monitoring are discussed below under Activity 8.

Illness in flocks, or the detection of an unusual or unexpected substance during routine monitoring for Class 1 and 2 substances, may be the only ways to detect potentially harmful levels of a Class 3 substance in feed and water. Routine monitoring for Class 3 substances is not appropriate, however, because of the enormous and ill-defined range of potential contaminants and the rarity with which any one of them will be present in sufficient quantities to pose a risk to public health. If a Class 3 contaminant is found, and if it cannot be determined whether its source was an accident that is not likely to be repeated, potentially affected feed or water should not be used until an adequate ongoing detection program is in place and an ADI or other long-term exposure limit is established.

Activity 6. Monitoring of Poultry Products

Careful sampling and analysis (monitoring) of feed and water is the most effective line of initial defense against contamination of poultry products but, as noted above, is not sufficient. The risk-management program must also include monitoring of poultry products themselves at a frequency and intensity that is matched to the magnitude of potential risk. Product monitoring is necessary for the following reasons:

- Monitoring of feed and water cannot be made 100% effective for any substance.
- The data necessary to establish appropriate feed and water tolerances are not available for many substances.
- For many chemicals, the relationship between feed and water levels and residue levels is not yet understood.
- Analytical methods have not been developed for some substances in feed or water.
- Class 3 substances may be easily overlooked in monitoring feed and water, or they may be encountered at other points in poultry production.

The intensity and frequency of product monitoring, and priorities assigned to such efforts, should be related to the effectiveness of the feed and water quality control. This is discussed further under Activity 8.

Product monitoring should ensure that poultry products containing residues above established tolerance limits for any of the three classes do not leave the processing plant if they ever enter it. However, there are practical limitations to the full realization of this objective, the principal one being that poultry cannot be held in storage during lengthy chemical analysis.

If poultry feed and water limits are properly set and enforced, there may still be occasional failures to keep residues within tolerance levels. These failures may have only limited health consequences, however, because tolerance limits for chronic exposure include large safety factors. Although there is no precise definition of an occasional failure, it should be assumed to mean rare occurrence in the life of an individual.

When such excursions above tolerance levels are detected, it should be determined whether they present any reason for concern about larger, longer, or more frequent violations of standards. Each such finding should trigger an effort to learn the cause of the problem and to find a remedy. In the context of adequate feed and water controls, it is not possible to predict how long such tolerance violations should be allowed to continue before poultry or poultry products are condemned. However, once a tolerance violation occurs, a risk assessment is needed at times to identify the seriousness of the potential risk. A decision could then be made on the need for condemnation as well as the need to change the feed and water tolerances, alter the production process, or intensify inspection.

Activity 7. Enforcement

Monitoring programs to manage risks are not effective unless they can ensure that excessively contaminated poultry feed or water is not used and that excessively contaminated poultry products do not reach consumers. Regulatory agencies have long had programs of enforcement to ensure that these objectives are met. The need for such programs is obvious, and no additional justification need be given here.

Activity 8. Establishing Priorities

Any program based on Activities 1 through 7 will require establishment of priorities. Two monitoring efforts (Activity 5, for feed and water, and Activity 6, for poultry products) require the development of sampling plans that can ensure, with some predetermined degree of confidence, that risk-management objectives are being achieved. As stated above, risk-management priorities and the frequency and intensity of monitoring should be based on risk assessment. For much risk-management planning, only the relative risks of various substances are of concern. A methodology for assessing relative risks is proposed in the following paragraphs.

Assessing Relative Risks

A scheme for assessing relative risks need not include estimation of the absolute risk of any of the substances to be ranked. It is necessary only that it incorporate in a systematic way some measures of both toxicity and exposure that are as accurate as possible; risk assessment cannot proceed without them. The exposure and toxicity data on Class 1, 2, and 3 chemicals vary widely in quality and content. These differences should be taken into account in a systematic way.

The primary purpose of a relative risk assessment is to ensure that the two major risk-management activities (monitoring of feed and water and monitoring of poultry products, including whole birds) achieve the intended objectives. That is, the degree of risk-management attention accorded a substance is directly related to the probability that it will be found in food intended for human consumption and to the risk it may pose if it escapes detection.

Two useful measures for ranking relative toxicity are the ADI (for noncarcinogens) and the UCR. These measures have the following desirable characteristics.

- They are derived from toxicity data in ways that are now rather well standardized and accepted.
- Different types of toxicity data gaps are treated in a relatively uniform way for different substances, e.g., by the application of standardized risk-assessment procedures.
- These measures are based on chronic exposure.
- They should be estimated for all substances monitored. (Recall that surveillance is used to identify substances for which risk assessment and tolerances need to be established, whereas monitoring is restricted to substances for which tolerances have been established.)

These two measures are adequate to rank the chronic toxicities of Class 1 and 2 substances. The committee knows of no other measures that have all the above characteristics.

To provide a systematic way of comparing carcinogens and noncarcinogens, it maybe necessary to develop a single toxicity scale that integrates both categories of substances. It is possible to derive an ADI equivalent for a carcinogen from its UCR by using certain assumptions about the level of risk considered to be negligible and the level of risk associated with an ADI for a threshold agent. Under the assumptions used to derive UCRs, carcinogens present a nonzero risk at all exposure levels above zero. Nevertheless, it is commonly accepted that for all carcinogens there is an exposure range that presents only a small risk, e.g., lifetime risks less than 10^{-5} or 10^{-6}, which reflect highly unlikely events.

It is not possible to demonstrate that an ADI carries absolutely no risk for the human population. At best, all that can be claimed for an ADI is that any potential risk is not likely to exceed some very small but quantified risk. In the absence of evidence to the contrary, and to provide two different toxicity scales for carcinogens and noncarcinogens, it may be assumed that the range of risk associated with an ADI is the same as that as that considered to be very small for carcinogens (i.e., 10^{-5} to 10^{-6}). This assumption is presented here only in the context of this specific risk-ranking objective to provide a systematic means for comparing the toxicities of carcinogens and noncarcinogens. It does not imply that the actual risk at an ADI is in the range assumed here.

It is further assumed that an ADI for a noncarcinogen will ensure that there is not more than a 10^{-6} (1 in a million) risk of a toxic effect occurring. An ADI equivalent derived for carcinogens will be taken as the dose estimated to give rise to the same maximum lifetime risk (10^{-6}). The ADI equivalents for carcinogens can then be directly compared to ADIs for noncarcinogens, because both will have been adjusted for potency and represent the same estimated risk level.

Figure 5-2 presents the linear low-dose response of several carcinogens with different UCRs. For each of these carcinogens, a dose providing an estimated lifetime risk of 10^{-6} can be identified. These ADI equivalents are represented by points for carcinogens A, B, C, and D along the dose scale. Thus, a carcinogen (B) with a UCR of 10^{-3} per unit of dose measured in mg/kg bw/day would have an ADI equivalent of 0.001 mg/kg/day. A UCR of 10^{-7} (carcinogen D) would correspond to an ADI equivalent of 10 mg/kg/day. These ADI equivalents can be calculated for the entire range of published UCRs. A representative range of ADIs and ADI equivalents and some possible toxicity ranking scores are presented in Table 5-3.

Unfortunately, there appears to be no single, direct measure of potential exposure. Thus, in constructing a ranking system for exposures, many factors must be considered. For example, the following factors all contribute to potential exposure for Class 1 and 2 substances:

1. The portion of the ADI or other tolerable limit to which people are ordinarily exposed. Frequent exposures to large fractions of the ADI (through poultry products only or through several environmental media) present higher potential risks than occasional exposures to only a small fraction of the ADI. A tolerance violation may have much greater significance for the former than for the latter exposure.
2. The frequency with which the chemical is or is likely to be detected in feed, water, or poultry products.
3. The volume of use for Class 1 substances and the volume of production, industrial use, or natural occurrence for Class 2 substances.
4. The number of birds treated or otherwise exposed.
5. The propensity for bioaccumulation.

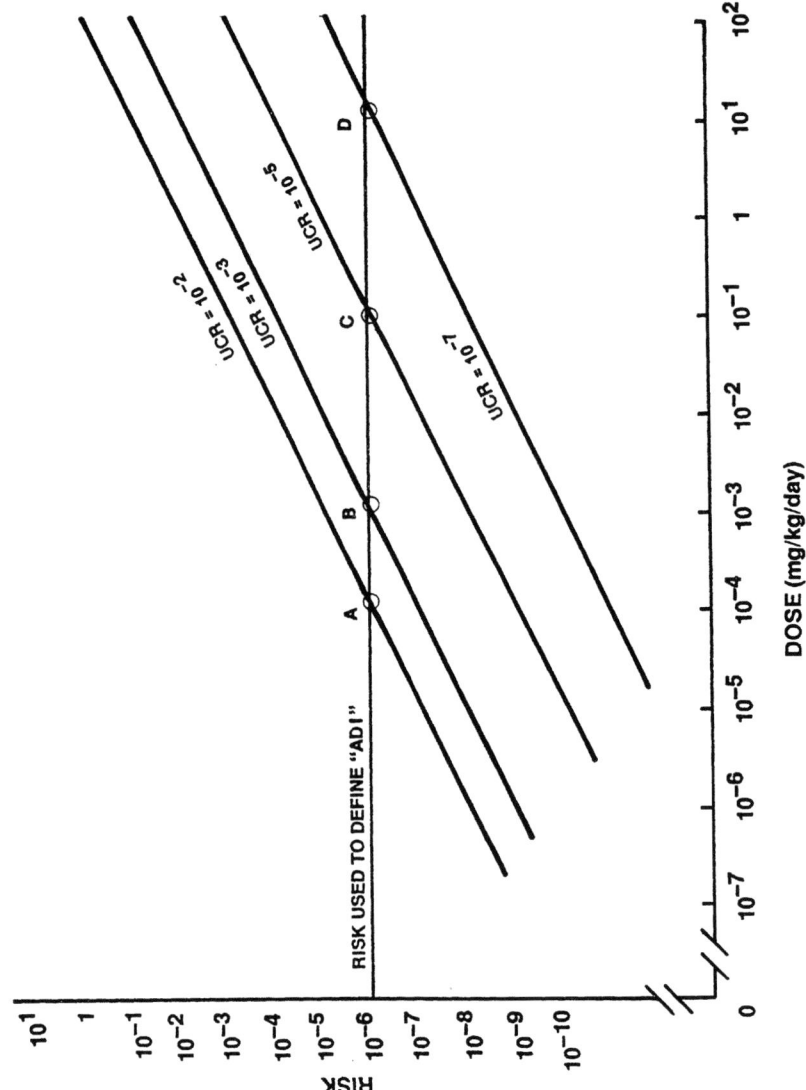

Figure 5-2
Derivation of ADI equivalents for carcinogens from UCR data. From Environ Corporation, 1985.

Table 5-3. Chronic Toxicity Scoring[a]

ADI Range (mg/kg/day)	Toxicity Score
$<10^{-7}$	9
$\geq 10^{-7} - <10^{-6}$	8
$\geq 10^{-6} - <10^{-5}$	7
$\geq 10^{-5} - <10^{-4}$	6
$\geq 10^{-4} - <10^{-3}$	5
$\geq 10^{-3} - <10^{-2}$	4
$\geq 10^{-2} - <10^{-1}$	3
$\geq 10^{-1} - <1$	2
≥ 1	1

[a] From Environ Corporation, 1985. For non-carcinogens, use ADI; for carcinogens, use an ADI equivalent, assuming a lifetime risk no greater than 10^{-6}.

6. The frequency and magnitude of consumption of the major tissues in which residues occur. (Substances accumulating in skin and muscle are of greater concern than those present only in the lung or kidney.)

FSIS should use these six factors to establish a ranking scheme for chemical exposures. Generally, the range of possible scores for potential exposure should approximately equal the range of toxicity scores (i.e., toxicity and exposure should be given approximately equal weight). One such scheme would be to assign a numeric score to each of the six items' for example, a score of 1 or 2 for factors 1 and 5; a score of 0, 1, or 2 for factor 3; and a score of 0, 2, or 4 for factors 2, 4, and 6. The total of these scores divided by 2 would yield exposure scores ranging from 1 through 9. The overall priority ranking system would then be based on a combination of this exposure score with the toxicity score.

Use of Relative Risk Scores. By systematic application of this ranking procedure, one should be able to establish priorities for monitoring feed, water, and poultry products and to develop sampling plans that are matched to the potential risks. The procedure should also be useful in establishing ADIs and tolerances for residue levels in poultry products.

Use of a single monitoring strategy for all chemicals would be inappropriate, since adequate attention would not be given to potentially high risk substances and too large a share of resources would be devoted to low risk substances. A more appropriate scheme would be based on first ranking the risk (e.g., high, medium, and low risk) and then categorizing the chemicals according to the type of risk they present (e.g., carcinogens, teratogens, liver toxicants). Intensive monitoring programs should be devised for potentially high-risk substances, less-intensive programs for those posing medium risks, and minimal monitoring activity for low-risk substances. Of course, ranking should be continually updated as new data emerge to determine the need for regrouping.

Of particular importance for the two-stage monitoring strategy described above is the choice of sampling rate. Statistical sampling strategies can be devised to ensure, with a specified degree of confidence, that products containing excessive levels of chemical residues are identified for removal from the food supply. The desirable degree of confidence for a potentially high-risk substance should be greater than for other substances. In Chapter 7, the committee recommends criteria for sampling chemical residues posing different levels of potential public health risk.

Finally, all eight essential activities of a risk-management program for chemical residues are based on applying, with varying degrees of rigor, the elements of a risk-assessment scheme based on specific types of data. Although an effective risk-management scheme will require all eight activities, not all of them need be under the direct control of FSIS. Indeed, some activities are already established at FDA and EPA. Nevertheless, to the extent possible, FSIS should ensure that all eight activities are under way and are adequately pursued.

SPECIAL PROBLEMS

As noted above, two aspects of chemical hazards in poultry require special treatment: Class 4 substances (those formed during processing, storing, and heating) and metabolites and degradation products of chemicals.

Class 4 Substances

The information needed to perform risk-assessment activities 1 through 3 for Class 4 substances is the same as that required for Classes 1, 2, and 3, but there are few data on the potential public health risks presented by these chemicals. For example, it appears that there has been no comprehensive risk assessment for any of these substances found in table-ready broiler chickens. Because Class 4 substances contaminate poultry products by mechanisms different from those for Classes 1, 2, and 3, it is not clear whether the risk-management strategies described for those classes are appropriate for Class 4. The committee believes it would be premature to devise a comprehensive risk-management strategy for them and recommends that FSIS initiate efforts to assess their risks in a comprehensive manner.

Metabolites and Degradation Products

In the regulation of residues in poultry, most attention has been given to the parent compounds administered to or ingested by the bird rather than to their metabolites or degradation products. EPA and FDA have given some consideration to those products, but it is not clear to the committee that the two agencies have treated the subject adequately or consistently.

There are no data indicating that metabolites or degradation products pose significant risks that are unregulated or that the risks of these products, to the extent they are considered, are under-or overestimated by the agencies. It nevertheless seems important to examine this issue carefully and to evaluate its present status.

ASSESSING PUBLIC HEALTH RISKS OF CHEMICAL RESIDUES IN POULTRY PRODUCTS

The magnitude of the public health risk from chemical residues in poultry products has not yet been examined, but the committee believes it important that such risk assessments be undertaken routinely. The chemical residue data developed by FSIS (Table 5-2) are not by themselves adequate for risk assessment, because the following information is lacking:

- the quantitative relationship between the levels of residues found in specific tissues examined by FSIS and the levels present in all other edible tissues;
- the amounts of different poultry products consumed by different segments of the population;
- the capability of the analytical methods used to detect residues below a certain level of contamination;
- toxicity data, ADIs, and UCRs for each residue;
- the level of human exposure resulting from other environmental media in which residues of the same chemicals may be present; and
- time trends in contamination patterns.

The information necessary to perform residue-specific risk assessments is available for many substances, especially those in Class 1. Access to FDA and EPA data files will be necessary to acquire the necessary toxicity and tissue distribution data and to estimate background levels. FSIS residue data should be analyzed statistically to determine the extent to which they are representative of the poultry product supply as a whole. These are tasks that can be completed with varying degrees of thoroughness for different residues. They should nevertheless be undertaken for all commonly found residues, but extreme care must be taken to ensure that the limitations in the data base and in the risk-assessment methodologies used are clearly set forth. Qualitative risk assessments should always be accompanied by descriptions of their limitations.

Because compliance with current tolerances for Class 1 chemicals is relatively high, it is likely that risk assessments undertaken for them will result in very low risk estimates. However, compliance with prescribed tolerances does not necessarily ensure low risk, since the adequacy of the data base for Class 1 substances has not been reviewed and there may be significant data gaps or limitations. Many substances in Class 1 were approved or registered by FDA and EPA many years ago; however, the committee knows of no routine federal effort to ensure that the data base for these substances meets current standards, except for limited EPA efforts with regard to some pesticides. It would thus be necessary to review the toxicity data base for Class 1 substances before accurate risk assessments can be completed.

The data base for Class 2 substances is certain to be less adequate than that for Class 1 substances. It is not even clear that all important chemicals in Class 2 have been identified. Nevertheless, risk assessment for Class 2 substances should be undertaken and limitations in data and methodology described to the extent possible with current information. It is particularly important to include information on other environmental sources of exposure to these chemicals, such as PCBs and some of the widely dispersed chlorinated hydrocarbon pesticides, so that the contribution of poultry products to total risk can be understood and the information can be used to establish special control programs where high risks exist and to reduce or eliminate programs now focusing on trivial problems. Although the committee examined the data and found no evidence of significant public health risks attributable to chemical residues in broilers, risk assessments and data are needed before definitive conclusions can be reached.

REFERENCES

Asher, I. M., and C. Zervos, eds. 1977. Structural Correlates of Carcinogenesis and Mutagenesis. A Guide to Testing Priorities? Proceedings of the Second FDA Office of Science Summer Symposium held at the U.S. Naval Academy, August 31-September 2, 1977. DHEW Publ. No. (FDA) 78-1046. The Office of Science, U.S. Food and Drug Administration, Rockville, Md. 241 pp.

Calabrese, E. J. 1983. Principles of Animal Extrapolation. Wiley, New York. 603 pp.

CFR (Code of Federal Regulations). 1986. Title 21, Food and Drugs; Section 520.2240a, Sulfaethoxypyridazine drinking water. U.S. Government Printing Office, Washington, D.C.

Doull, J., C. D. Klaassen, and M. O. Amdur, eds. 1980. Casarett and Doull's Toxicology—The Basic Science of Poisons, 2nd ed. Macmillan, New York. 778 pp.

Environ Corporation. 1985. Documentation for the Development of Toxicity and Volume Scores for the Purpose of Scheduling Hazardous Wastes. Prepared for the Office of Solid Waste, U.S. Environmental Protection Agency. EPA Contract No. 68-01-6861, Subcontract No. 38-9. Environ Corporation, Washington, D.C. 130 pp.

EPA (Environmental Protection Agency). 1980. Water quality criteria documents; availability. Notice of water quality criteria documents. Fed. Regist. 45:79317-79379.

EPA (Environmental Protection Agency). 1982. Pesticide Assessment Guidelines, Subdivision F, Hazard Evaluation: Human and Domestic Animals. Publ. No. EPA 540/9-82-025. Office of Pesticide Programs, Office of Pesticides and Toxic Substances, U.S. Environmental Protection Agency, Washington, D.C. 163 pp. Available from the National Technical Information Service in Springfield, Va., as PB83-153916.

EPA (Environmental Protection Agency). 1985. Health Assessment Document for Chloroform: Final Report. Publ. No. EPA/600/8-84/004F. Office of Health and Environmental Assessment, U.S. Environmental Protection Agency, Washington, D.C. [415 pp.] Available from the National Technical Information Service in Springfield, Va., as PB86-105004.

FDA (Food and Drug Administration). 1979. Polychlorinated biphenyls (PCB's); reduction of tolerances. Final rule. Docket No. 77N-0080. Fed. Regist. 44:38330-38340.

FDA (Food and Drug Administration). 1982a. D&C Green No. 6; listing as a color additive in externally applied drugs and cosmetics. Final rule. Docket No. 81N-0301. Fed. Regist. 47:14138-14147.

FDA (Food and Drug Administration). 1982b. Toxicological Principles for the Safety Assessment of Direct Food Additives and Color Additives Used in Food. Bureau of Foods, U.S. Food and Drug Administration, Washington, D.C. [248 pp.]

FDA (Food and Drug Administration). 1985. Sponsored compounds in food producing animals; criteria and procedures for evaluating the safety of carcinogenic residues. Proposed rule. Docket No. 77N-0026. Fed. Regist. 50:45530-45555.

FSC (Food Safety Council). 1980. Proposed System for Food Safety Assessment. Final Report of the Scientific Committee of the Food Safety Council. Food Safety Council, Washington, D.C. 160 pp.

Klaassen, C. D., and J. Doull. 1980. Evaluation of safety: Toxicologic evaluation. Pp. 11-27 in J. Doull, C. D. Klaassen, and M. O. Amdur, eds. Casarett and Doull's Toxicology—The Basic Science of Poisons, 2nd ed. Macmillan, New York.

Lehman, A. J., and O. G. Fitzhugh. 1954. 100-fold margin of safety. Assoc. Food Drug Off., Q. Bull. 18:33-35.

Loomis, T. A. 1978. Essentials of Toxicology, 3rd ed. Lea & Febiger, Philadelphia. 245 pp.

MacMahon, B., and T. F. Pugh. 1970. Epidemiology: Principles and Methods. Little, Brown, Boston. 376 pp.

Nisbet, I. C. T. 1981. The role of exposure assessment in risk evaluation: Research needs. Pp. 419-429 in C. R. Richmond, P. J. Walsh, and E. D. Copenhaver, eds. Health Risk Analysis, Proceedings of the Third Life Sciences Symposium. Franklin Institute Press, Philadelphia.

NRC (National Research Council). 1977. Drinking Water and Health. Report of the Safe Drinking Water Committee, Advisory Center on Toxicology. National Academy of Sciences, Washington, D.C. 939 pp.

NRC (National Research Council). 1980a. Drinking Water and Health, Vol. 3. Report of the Safe Drinking Water Committee, Board on Toxicology and Environmental Health Hazards. National Academy Press, Washington, D.C. 415 pp.

NRC (National Research Council). 1980b. Risk Assessment/Safety Evaluation of Food Chemicals. Report of the Subcommittee on Food Toxicology, Committee on Food Protection, Food and Nutrition Board. National Academy Press, Washington, D.C. 36 pp.

NRC (National Research Council). 1983. Risk Assessement in the Federal Government: Managing the Process. Report of the Committee on the Institutional Means for Assessment of Risks to Public Health, Commission on Life Sciences. National Academy Press, Washington, D.C. 203 pp.

NRC (National Research Council). 1984. Toxicity Testing, Strategies to Determine Needs and Priorities. Report of the Steering Committee on Identification of Toxic and Potentially Toxic Chemicals for Consideration by the National Toxicology Program, Board on Toxicology and Environmental Health Hazards. National Academy Press, Washington, D.C. 395 pp.

NRC (National Research Council). 1985. Meat and Poultry Inspection: The Scientific Basis of the Nation's Program. Report of the Committee on the Scientific Basis of the Nation's Meat and Poultry Inspection Program, Food and Nutrition Board. National Academy Press, Washington, D.C. 209 pp.

NRC (National Research Council). 1986. Drinking Water and Health, Vol. 6. Report of the Safe Drinking Water Committee, Board on Toxicology and Environmental Health Hazards. National Academy Press, Washington, D.C. 457 pp.

OSTP (Office of Science and Technology Policy). 1985. Chemical carcinogens; a review of the science and its associated principles, February 1985. Final document. Fed. Regist. 50:10372-10442.

Rodricks, J., and M. R. Taylor. 1983. Application of risk assessment to food safety decision making. Regul. Toxicol. Pharmacol. 3:275-307.

Chapter 6

Application of the Model to the Current FSIS Inspection System

In evaluating the current FSIS poultry inspection program, the committee identified those parts of poultry production, slaughtering, and processing that appear to present the greatest risk to public health, especially in terms of microbial and chemical contamination. Current FSIS inspection activities were then compared with those risks to determine whether the methods used are appropriate for detecting and preventing risk, to identify areas in which major risks seem to be inadequately addressed, and to determine where current or proposed inspection practices seem to provide little protection for public health.

The committee's findings are discussed below according to the major component of the risk model to which they apply.

THE POULTRY PRODUCTION SUBMODEL

Breeding

With help from the U.S. agricultural research system, the poultry industry has made substantial progress in improving management practices and the genetic quality of broilers. As a result, the incidence of economically important diseases has been sharply reduced in the broiler population over the last 40 years. However, some disadvantages indirectly accompany the benefits derived from standardization of the genetic base and the development of mass production practices in the broiler industry. In particular, diseases in broiler houses can be economically disastrous because of the high-density holding of genetically homogeneous groups of animals that are uniformly susceptible to diseases (Crittenden, 1979; Fenner et al., 1974). Poultry producers tend to use prophylactic drugs to minimize the probability of economically ruinous disease outbreaks, thereby setting the stage for potential human health problems from drug residues and from resistant strains of bacteria (Harris et al., 1986; Holmberg et al., 1984; NRC, 1979, 1980).

The Food Safety and Inspection Service (FSIS) has no legal authority or responsibility to monitor the genetic stock or the breeding process, although other parts of the U.S. Department of

Agriculture (USDA), notably the Cooperative State Research Service and the Agricultural Research Service, fund important poultry science programs. Because of the indirect connection between the genetic makeup of poultry stock and the public health hazards noted above, it would be useful for those responsible for product safety in FSIS to maintain closer communication with those involved in research on poultry genetics, e.g., poultry science departments at land grant colleges, the Agricultural Research Service, and the poultry industry. FSIS should also be in a position to work closely with poultry science laboratories as new research programs are considered, undertaken, and tested in the field.

Hatching

Infectious agents can contaminate poultry during hatching. Organisms such as Mycoplasma and Salmonella may infect chicks prior to hatching if infected breeders transmit them transovarially, thus providing a focus of infection for the flock in the grow-out house. Egg-shell contamination by Aspergillus, E. coli, and Salmonella can also contaminate the hatcher and conveyor belts used to transfer chicks from the hatcher through vaccination and sorting to crating for transfer to the grow-out house. Some forms of Salmonella have been associated with systemic disease in chicks less than 3 weeks old (Cruickshank et al., 1982), and avian leukosis viruses (ALV) have been observed in chicken embryos (Crittenden, 1979; Fenner et al., 1974). Although ALV has not been associated with diseases that can be transmitted to humans, the natural history of bird-to-bird transmission of this virus shows that the hatching stage of this submodel is a potentially susceptible critical control point with regard to human health.

Grow-Out

The possible introduction of microbial hazards, such as Salmonella, and chemical hazards, such as chlorinated hydrocarbon pesticides, are major concerns during the grow-out phase. A variety of infectious microorganisms known to be pathogenic in humans can grow, multiply, and spread undetected among the chickens in the grow-out house. Pesticides, drugs, and other chemicals introduced in low concentrations can become highly concentrated in the tissues of the birds.

Sanitation

Sanitation controls are important in all phases of poultry production (breeding, hatching, grow-out), since most pathogens of concern are exogenous to the broiler stock. Broilers are most often born healthy and substantially free of contamination. It is primarily in the grow-out environment that pathogens, residues, and diseases may be introduced. FSIS has no control over the level of sanitation at grow-out facilities, but because of the economic incentives of growing healthy birds, almost all major manufacturers (accounting for more than 90% of the young chickens produced in the United States) follow good sanitation practices.

From a health perspective, disease outbreaks are sometimes so disastrous that entire flocks are lost or must be destroyed. FSIS must ensure that condemned birds are indeed destroyed and do not reappear at the slaughter house for processing.

Feed Milling and Feed Protection

Young chickens intended to be grown and slaughtered within 3 months after birth are fed highly enriched diets. During this period, three potential public health risks are presented: unintentional contamination of feed or water with natural toxins, drugs, or other chemicals; inadequate withdrawal from drugs intentionally added to feed; and microbial contamination of feed.

Unintentional drug contamination of feed can occur during commercial feed production and milling, which are largely decentralized. The cleanliness of feed mills and the technology used in them can affect the health of young broilers. Unintentional mixing of feeds and raw materials intended for diverse purposes may occur because one plant may oversee the manufacture of many products. This environment provides the opportunity for cross-contamination of feed components. Drugs and vitamins are often added, and if residues are not adequately removed from the mill after a mix, substantial drug contamination of the following batch can occur. The feed constituents themselves can also be contaminated with pesticides or other environmental chemicals.

It is recognized that feed mill contamination is a potential human health problem. Thus, all mills are theoretically regulated and inspected by the Food and Drug Administration (FDA). In practice, however, only a small percentage (e.g., 25-33%) of the feed mills in question are inspected each year because of constraints on FDA resources. FSIS relies entirely on FDA to monitor feed mill contamination. Because of the limited resources at both FDA and the FSIS National Residue Program (NRP), one can reasonably ask whether the level of protection is sufficient.

Certain FDA-approved drugs (e.g., antibiotics and coccidiostats) are deliberately added to poultry feed during milling to prevent poultry diseases or to promote growth. Most of these drugs are not used to treat disease in humans, but each of them has designated withdrawal times, i.e., the amount of time prior to slaughter during which the drug is not to be used to prevent unsafe residues of the drugs from contaminating edible tissues. These withdrawal times are important, because drugs and residues can have potentially adverse effects on consumers (Settepani, 1984).

FDA, which has its own resource constraints, is responsible for ensuring that the presence of approved animal drugs is monitored by acceptable analytic methods and that there is adherence to specified withdrawal times. USDA's Animal and Plant Health Inspection Service (APHIS) assumes some responsibility for working with FDA because of its responsibility to prevent animal disease. This is an area requiring collaboration between FSIS, APHIS, and FDA personnel, but progress is sometimes limited by legitimate disagreements on technical problems. For example, attempts to agree on uniform analytical methods used to detect drug contamination of feeds have been hampered by disagreements over which method is best. In addition, it has been difficult to agree on the amount of resources devoted to monitoring and testing.

Poultry feed given to broiler flocks has been demonstrated to be a source of salmonellae that subsequently contaminate broiler carcasses (Williams, 1981). Thus, FSIS should investigate further the possibility of providing Salmonella-free feed for broilers. FSIS authority over Salmonella contamination of broiler carcasses is presently restricted to critical control points during slaughtering and processing, but greater protection of public health might result if attention were given to the points at which Salmonella is introduced during production, beginning with the introduction of Salmonella into feed (see also Chapter 4).

Until reliably Salmonella-free feed ingredients can be ensured, the poultry industry should consider restricting its feed supply to pelleted material, which reduces the potential for Salmonella contamination (Shapcott, 1985). When feed is processed at 180°F (82.22°C) or higher, levels of microbial contamination are effectively reduced. However, this process alone will not guarantee a Salmonella-free product (Blankenship et al., 1985; Cover et al., 1985), and efforts should continue to be made to reduce the level of contamination at each critical control point during the manufacture of feed and feed ingredients and in feeding processes and equipment within the production submodel.

Natural Toxicants and Other Environmental Contaminants

Contamination of groundwater supplies by environmental contaminants has generated concerns about chemical contamination of water used in poultry production and slaughter. For example, chlorinated hydrocarbon pesticides maybe used in fields near grow-out houses, and safeguards must be (and are) taken to protect against the accidental contamination of poultry feed during grow-out. Air pollution is another problem in some settings, and care must be given to air-filtering systems, which are sometimes used by growers.

In all these cases, the possibility of serious accidental contamination by environmental contaminants is minimized by the integrated structure of the poultry industry. This structure facilitates self-monitoring and communication of potential problems between subcomponents of the production phase. There is an increasingly strong capability along with a financial incentive to trace flocks back through the production system to determine the causes of specific problems and to ensure that the production of unfit animals is rapidly terminated.

To assist farmers in developing adequate production practices, the FSIS transferred $3 million to the USDA Cooperative Extension Service over a 3-year period from 1983 to 1985. In turn, this service has provided funds to state extension services for programs to teach farmers about the appropriate use of chemicals and drugs and to provide information about the overall production environment. Intuitively, this cooperative effort seems reasonable, but it would be useful to evaluate its effect on overall risk in poultry production.

Important microbial and chemical risks occur during poultry production, but FSIS must rely extensively on economic incentives to growers and on the often uncoordinated efforts of other federal and state agencies for which food safety is not a primary objective. FSIS's lack of authority to control the front end of the production process (i.e., the raw materials used in production) increases the importance of FSIS inspection activities once young birds enter the slaughterhouses.

Transit

Poultry are most often transported from grow-out houses to slaughtering facilities on trucks. During transport, susceptible or poorly protected birds are subjected to great stress, and deaths are not uncommon. This phase also provides a major opportunity for unscrupulous operators to reintroduce dead, diseased, or dying birds into the human food chain. Care must be taken to ensure that raw material destined for pet food, for example, is not reintroduced into food being produced for human consumption. None of this generally has much implication for human health, but it brings to light some issues to be considered in attempts to ensure that wholesome food is placed on the consumer's plate. FSIS employs several dozen compliance officers who visit production facilities throughout the country searching for such potential health-related factors as problems in transit.

SLAUGHTERING SUBMODEL

FSIS responsibilities for poultry inspection begin at the gate of the slaughterhouses. As the trucks roll in carrying the broilers in holding crates, federal authority passes to FSIS from a variety of other agencies (e.g., state agriculture departments, APHIS, EPA, and FDA). Sometimes the inspectors on site will know from experience what to expect from the animals supplied by a particular farm or grow-out house. Often they will have been stationed at the same plant for an extended period or they will themselves live nearby and thus will know something about both the grower and any recent environmental conditions or diseases in the area. Frequently, however, they will have neither formal information about disease incidence in the bird population nor a systematic way of evaluating the health of the birds other than by visual inspection. The growers are concerned about the health of their flocks during grow-out and transit, but they have strong disincentives to provide any information that can be used against them at later stages. Similarly, plant personnel are not particularly forthcoming about problems. Moreover, no other state or federal agency is required to provide FSIS with such information. Accordingly, FSIS inspectors pursue this responsibility essentially without assistance.

Antemortem Inspection

In this highly informal, unsystematic environment, the inspection staff begins its first task, antemortem inspection. Birds may be examined while they are still in cages on trucks so that a subjective determination can be made about the overall condition of the flock. As the thousands of birds are pulled out and placed on a line, the inspector makes a rough visual determination of the prevalence of disease in the flock. Years ago, when birds were slaughtered by the dozens or hundreds, this procedure was more effective than it is now when as many as 60,000-70,000 birds (depending on line speed) pass through antemortem inspection daily.

From an aesthetic and public health perspective, this inspection appears to detect little. Perhaps one plus is that the resources required to conduct antemortem inspection are very small.

Approval of Slaughtering Facilities

Before a slaughtering facility can begin operation, blueprints for the plant must be approved by FSIS (CFR, 1986a). This practice was adopted in the 1950s, apparently to ensure that proper water supplies were available to the plant (e.g., that sewage and freshwater supplies would not be mixed) and that materials in the plant would not be good breeding grounds for microbial organisms. The necessity for approval of blueprints should be continually reevaluated, along with other steps in the overall inspection strategy, as FSIS constantly shifts resources to match them with evolving hazards.

Current rules require that an inspector examine slaughterhouses every morning before operations begin (USDA, 1983a). During this procedure, the inspector must ensure that all work surfaces are clean to the naked eye, that temperatures are within required ranges (e.g., in scalders and chillers), that condensation in cooled areas is minimal, that no illegal chemicals are on the premises, and that lines are operating properly and are well lighted. This inspection can be a helpful quality assurance technique if properly conducted. Although many potential health problems are not visible to the naked eye, the requirements for visible cleanliness probably helps to ensure adequate public health protection.

Stun, Scald, and Pluck

FSIS participates little in the development of technology for this part of the process, although new equipment and techniques could have an impact on carcass contamination.

Evisceration and Postmortem Inspection

FSIS plays a major role in the evisceration and postmortem inspection of poultry. It is an important responsibility, since these procedures provide almost a single line of defense against the intrusion of pathogens into the food supply.

Following is a list of the key variables in the evisceration and postmortem inspection process:

- Quality of the mechanical devices and procedures used in evisceration.
- Placement of the viscera next to the bird of origin to facilitate matching of the two.
- Inspection time (line speed).
- Quality of the postmortem inspection procedure.
- Quality assurance techniques.

Quality of the Mechanical Devices and Procedures Used in Evisceration. The greatest risk of microbial contamination is presented when the gastrointestinal tract is separated from the rest of the carcass. Ideally, this process should be designed to decrease or eliminate fecal contamination and cross-contamination. Current practices do not achieve this goal, however, despite the introduction of automatic evisceration machines in the mid-to late 1970s that facilitated the inspection of entrails and observation of the open body cavity. The new equipment often malfunctions, resulting in poor placement of the carcass, and the gastrointestinal tracts are frequently broken so that feces and other intestinal contents contaminate the surface of the birds with a variety of bacteria, including salmonellae. Decreased line speeds might eliminate many of these shortcomings, but such speeds would have to be substantially slower than those used in traditional inspection.

Placement of the Intestinal Tract. Carcass evisceration facilitates the inspection process by enabling the inspectors to obtain a clear view of the viscera of each bird while enabling them to associate the viscera (including heart, liver, and spleen) with the carcass to which they belong and thus to prevent contamination and cross-contamination between diseased and healthy carcasses or viscera. The current poultry processing system and the inspection system seem to accomplish this well.

Inspection Time (Line Speed). Once the carcass has been eviscerated, and the carcass and viscera have either been separated (but tagged for identification) or hung together for easy viewing, the bird approaches the inspectors. Depending on the line speeds in the Streamlined Inspection System (SIS) and the New Line speed (NELS) system, the inspector has between 1 and 1.5 seconds to perform the entire postmortem inspection, and that time is further decreased in the Third-Generation System, in which one inspector would be responsible for 180 birds per minute. It appears that little attempt has been made to evaluate inspection methods and line speeds with regard to fecal contamination, microbiological quality, and public health impact. Over the past decade FSIS has spent a substantial amount of time investigating the effects of accelerated line speed on inspection and trying to devise work measurement standards that would enable one or more inspectors to conduct postmortem inspection more rapidly. If these rapid line speeds can be shown to result in greater fecal contamination, a case might be made for slowing the process, even though substantial contamination may also occur in other ways (such as in the chiller) and despite the fact that we cannot relate the exact load of bacteria on birds at this stage to the load present on the consumer's dinner plate.

Numerous microbiological surveys of consumer-ready poultry have demonstrated that many carcasses are heavily contaminated with fecal flora, even when the carcasses are clean to the naked eye, but this contamination may not be associated with line speed. Surveys of 15 federally inspected plants conducted in 1967 and 1979—before line speeds were accelerated—determined the incidence of salmonellae in processed, ready-to-market, whole young chickens (Green et al., 1982). In the 1967 study, salmonellae were isolated from 28.6% (mean) of the chickens; in 1979, 36.9% of similarly analyzed chicken samples were positive. A more recent 2-year survey of the same 15 plants conducted from 1982 to 1984—after poultry line speeds were increased—revealed that 35% were positive for salmonellae (R. W. Johnston, FSIS, personal communication, 1986). Before it can be stated with assurance that line speed is irrelevant from a public health perspective, more studies on this subject need to be conducted. Current evidence seems to indicate, however, that the mix of changing conditions in production and slaughter—including accelerated line speeds—results in a product that is not contaminated more often than it was before line speeds were increased.

Quality of the Postmortem Inspection Procedure. Bird-by-bird postmortem inspection as described in Chapters 2 and 3 is required for all poultry slaughtered in an FSIS-inspected establishment. To ensure that the postmortem inspection proceeds effectively, FSIS requires plants to provide some form of control (e.g., a switch or button) so that the inspectors can stop, start, or slow the lines on which the birds are hung. Adequate lighting of uniform intensity at all work levels is also required. Double lines must be separated by dividers to prevent confusion and to ensure that each carcass receives the inspector's attention, and as indicated above, visceral organs must be kept with the carcass from which they have been removed. Hand-washing facilities must be adequate and properly located at both operating and inspection positions (Libby, 1975).

Trained company employees are assigned to each inspector to perform such functions as picking feathers, trimming bruises, moving condemned birds from the lines into condemned cans, placing suspect birds on racks for more detailed inspection, marking the condemnation record sheets, and generally assisting the inspector in tasks related to inspection procedures.

The objectives of each of the postmortem inspection techniques described in Chapter 2 are to ensure that no visible lesions or systemic infections reach the consumer in either whole birds or parts of birds. The inspection procedures do not have as their objectives the diagnoses of any specific disease state that could be transmitted from broilers to humans. Under any form of manual inspection, including traditional, modified traditional, hands on/hands off, new line speed, or streamlined inspection system, there are ample opportunities for microbial contamination to spread from carcass to carcass. Moreover, there is no provision for making a systematic examination to determine the presence of chemical residues, including drugs and environmental contaminants. Thus, the weight of the evidence suggests that the current program is not effectively protecting the public health. The committee believes that whatever benefits the current system may provide, the alternative strategies discussed in Chapter 7, including detailed inspection of a sample of birds, may provide greater public health protection. Accordingly, FSIS should strongly consider immediate changes in its current inspection practices.

If substantial public resources are to continue to be dedicated to bird-by-bird poultry inspection as it is currently conducted even under the most streamlined circumstances, it is important for FSIS to demonstrate the associated public health benefits, if any, as soon as possible. If aesthetic improvements are the only benefits derived from the present system, the committee believes there is no justification for continuing the government's intense involvement.

Quality Assurance Techniques. In the current inspection system, condemned whole carcasses are discarded and are thus highly unlikely to reenter the food chain. However, since some birds that should be condemned are passed, and since the link between carcasses and the viscera is lost once the parts have passed the postmortem inspection station, there is substantial likelihood that contaminated parts are brought together with clean parts on a regular basis.

After evaluating each part of the evisceration and postmortem procedure, the committee came to the following conclusions:

- FSIS should continue to apply substantial resources to this part of the production system, especially because of the absence of safeguards in poultry production, but these resources should be better justified and reallocated in ways more likely to protect the public health.
- The public health impact of resources applied to this part of the production system need to be evaluated.
- FSIS should conduct further studies to determine the impact of inspection line speed on public health.

Chemical Traceback

The U.S. poultry industry is highly integrated, with strong relationships extending from producer to wholesaler. Accordingly, unlike most of the red meat industry, there is a substantial capability to trace known episodes of contamination back through the system to their sources. This traceback capability, along with producer education, probably decreases the risk from chemical contamination in the poultry supply. So do the economic and public relations repercussions of major recalls; several widely publicized incidents during the late 1970s also impressed upon poultry producers the unpleasant consequences of serious lapses (USDA, 1980).

National Residue Program

Monitoring. The number of samples tested in the National Residue Program (NRP) is designed to ensure, at a 95% confidence level, that a chemical will be detected in at least one sample, if it occurs with a uniform distribution in 1% or more of the population of birds or animals slaughtered each year (USDA, 1983b, c, 1984, 1985a). Since more than 4 billion broilers are slaughtered annually, as many as 40 million broilers could be contaminated without detection by the current inspection system. Thus, the chance of any animal being sampled in the United States is minuscule. This is not adequate for effective public health protection. Because hazards are not uniformly distributed over populations of poultry or consumers, this overall contamination rate of 1% could represent a substantial public health hazard to normal as well as highly susceptible persons.

Thus, FSIS should consider revising its sampling program. Following are some of the technical problems and opportunities that will need to be weighed:

- Ensuring randomness, so that neither inspectors nor plant personnel can forecast which items are to be sampled and no element of personal discretion affects sample selection. This may be an especially important consideration in sampling birds on the line.
- Due consideration of alternatives to simple random sampling to meet program objectives by using the smallest possible samples and to minimize complexity in interpretation. For example, there will be good reasons to sample at different rates under

different circumstances. Stratified random sampling may have many advantages.

- Selecting the percentage of birds to be sampled and changing those percentages as new data indicate local or widespread short-or long-term variations in the likelihood of finding significant risks to health. For example, it may be desirable to increase the percentage of birds sampled even up to 100% (the present approach to organoleptic inspection) when observations indicate that a particular flock presents health risks not adequately controlled by plant personnel in their own inspections. This might occur when many of the birds are septicemic, when evisceration equipment is out of adjustment, or when a sampled bird dies from causes other than slaughter.
- Calculating variances correctly for use with quantitative estimates based on data from complex samples.

The committee believes that a two-stage sampling scheme, with a third stage for more detailed examination, may be best for the inspection of whole slaughtered birds. This system is described in Chapter 7.

Surveillance Testing. FSIS continues to develop new methods to enable it to test for residues more rapidly, perhaps while carcasses are still in the plant. However, no new tests for environmental contaminants of poultry have been brought on line.

The committee concluded that sample size in the FSIS surveillance program is not adequate, and that its tie with the monitoring program ensures that it cannot be truly representative of the residue problem in the broiler population.

Exploratory Testing. The committee reviewed the current exploratory testing program and found that existing methods of selecting samples and determining sampling frequency are inadequate. Furthermore, it believes that FSIS does not rigorously follow the eight steps described in Chapter 5 that are needed for an effective residue control program. In particular, the committee concluded that FSIS should play a larger role in determining the degree of consumer exposure to various agents that might be found in poultry and that the current FSIS program is not adequate to deal with occasional but potentially serious contamination.

Operations. In the NRP, an inspector in charge, usually a veterinarian, receives a computer print-out specifying the number of carcasses to be sampled and a sampling plan for collecting those carcasses. Each plant makes provisions for collecting, labeling, freezing, and transporting the requested samples to one of FSIS's national laboratories, where they wait in a queue for analysis.

As many as 10 days may elapse before results are reported. The effective communication of results requires vigilance from a supervisor and good mechanisms for communicating between the field and headquarters in Washington, D.C. Once a report arrives at headquarters, information must be relayed across program lines from the Deputy Administrator for Science to field operations. Any problems must be further communicated to the employees and FSIS compliance staff at the plant.

This system is both cumbersome and slow when it works as planned, and there are many opportunities for further delays and complete breakdowns. FSIS established mechanisms for minimizing delays after a serious problem occurred in Montana in 1979 (USDA, 1980), but even under good circumstances, a month can pass before contamination found in the system is brought to the attention of administrative officials and action can be taken. As stated before in the discussion on monitoring, the odds of catching even continuous but not nationwide contamination, should it exist, are very low. Many years could go by before even one bird from a given plant is sampled and the process of analysis and notification can begin.

Several reforms could speed this process. In particular, the time required to store and transport samples to FSIS laboratories could be shortened, and new resources could be devoted to speeding up laboratory testing and the communication of results. A relatively small infusion of laboratory and testing resources could improve methodology, substantially shorten the queue, speed the development of methodology, and enhance the strength of the program.

Washing and Chilling to Inhibit Microbial Growth

Questions have been raised about the safety of communal ice baths because of the potential for microbial contamination to spread among the thousands of carcasses immersed in the same tank. In the absence of adequate data, it is not clear to the committee that so-called dry chill procedures are inherently better in reducing overall bacterial contamination. The committee urges FSIS to collect more data to support a thorough comparison of chill procedures.

Following chilling, the birds are reinspected to check for the presence of defects, according to recently adopted finished product standards. Birds not meeting these standards will be classified as adulterated (Anonymous, 1986).

Less than 1% of birds inspected are condemned, according to current criteria (see Table 2-2 in Chapter 2) (USDA, 1985b). A large portion of the birds carry undetected enteric bacteria that are harmful to humans. Some of these bacteria may have been introduced by the process of poultry inspection itself. A smaller number of birds contain drug or pesticide residues that exceed prescribed limits. Such problems can persist for some time in the current inspection system before action is taken, and postmortem inspection itself may have little direct effect on them.

THE PACKING AND PROCESSING SUBMODEL

Most young chickens are sent directly to market, but an increasingly larger percentage of them are being processed further in response to consumer demand for more ready-to-eat food and food that requires less preparation time. Some of the risks to human health introduced during this processing are described in Chapter 4. After reviewing the data, the committee concluded that the risks presented during packing and processing are managed quite adequately.

Further processing includes cutting up whole chickens and packaging the pieces. The pieces are often obtained from birds that when whole are not aesthetically acceptable. At this stage, microbial contamination may be introduced by cutting boards and saws that are not adequately cleaned.

Both regulation and technology seem to be adequate to deal with the major potential health hazards that arise when cooking is part of further processing. The consequences of improper cooking could be disastrous for manufacturers, so they will go to great lengths to avoid errors. Once optimal cooking conditions have been determined, it would not be difficult to ensure that the cooking time and the temperature are adequate through monitoring.

Hazards presented by food additives during the packing and preparation of poultry are described in Chapter 3 (pp. 41-42). FDA is responsible for setting standards for food additives, and FSIS evaluates the specific use of each additive in poultry products. Although there may be some marginal benefits to this reevaluation by FSIS, it is difficult to justify duplication of a process to which the FDA devotes major scientific and financial resources.

Evaluation of potential risks from packing material is complex; it includes the identification, measurement, and toxicological evaluation of compounds obtained from the material under various storage conditions. Although there is no information directly linking the small amounts of these compounds that may be present in foods to adverse effects on human health, FDA approval is required for all materials used to package poultry in the United States (Karel and Heidelbaugh, 1975; Sacharow, 1979).

Quality assurance has progressed rapidly in the entire poultry processing industry. This change is not altruistic; more and more managers understand the necessity to keep their production systems under control for financial and regulatory reasons.

FSIS has historically provided daily inspection of processing as it is required to do for slaughtering. Inspectors look for a variety of regulatory violations in an attempt to police the industry. In the past, some plant managers have looked upon the inspection service as a substitute for having their own quality assurance program. Since 1980, FSIS has encouraged the development of voluntary quality control systems in plants. These systems are designed to emphasize good manufacturing and control practices and to provide both the manufacturer and the FSIS inspection staff with a more systematic look at the production process. The NRC report on meat and poultry inspection (NRC, 1985) described some successes and shortcomings of this system.

DISTRIBUTION AND PREPARATION SUBMODEL

Transport to Retailer

Once a product leaves the plant in either fresh or processed form, the federal government has no more control over it. In extreme circumstances, FSIS can use plant records to locate shipments in warehouses or supermarkets before the product reaches the consumer. FSIS has the power to impound the product, pending the outcome of an administrative or judicial process.

The time it takes for fresh products to be transported from the plant to the supermarket is, on average, only several days and can be as short as 1 day. During this period the product is once more at risk but is not subject to regulation by FSIS or any other federal agency.

Handling in the Retail System

At retail, many poultry products bear a label identifying the manufacturer. Accordingly, consumers do not regard such products as a general commodity as they do red meat, but, rather, as a product of the specified brand-name producer. This labeling provides manufacturers with an incentive to make high quality products available to consumers in return for a premium price. In addition, large poultry chains, wholesalers, and retail store managers have an economic incentive to ensure the adequacy of environmental conditions inside the retail store and to prevent spoilage or contamination beyond that already on the product when it enters the store.

The Multiple Roles of Labeling

Every manufacturer must label each product to show its ingredients. Nutritional labeling is optional, but if done, must conform to specific guidelines (CFR, 1986b). Labels may also suggest proper modes of preparation and provide recipes. Such information is provided at the discretion of the manufacturer and is not subject to FSIS approval unless it impinges on other regulated issues, e.g., the rank order of ingredients, net weight, or the size of type specified for some required information.

There are no systematic efforts to educate consumers about the possible dangers of mishandling or improperly cooking poultry products. FSIS offers some educational information about food safety through a variety of public affairs programs, including school poster contests, public service spots on radio and television, and consumer hot-lines. These programs should be emphasized and broadened, since the major role of improper food handling in disease outbreaks has been well documented (Bryan, 1978, 1980). Therefore, the probability is high that morbidity rates can be controlled effectively through consumer education and action.

Accordingly, any rational risk-management strategy to combat enteric diseases derived from poultry must include a substantially stronger informational component than presently exists. At minimum the committee suggests that simple labels be attached to each ready-to-cook bird to remind consumers about the preparation procedures that are necessary to avoid illness. Such labeling need not encourage consumers to avoid the product. Rather, a simple tag emphasizing the need to wash all implements, cook the product thoroughly, and chill leftovers as soon possible after serving could go a long way toward adequate consumer protection. FSIS should use its existing authority or seek additional authority, if necessary, to implement such a system if it is unable to persuade manufacturers to label their products voluntarily. Such a labeling system should not be regarded as a substitute for other attempts by FSIS and industry to reduce the overall load of bacteria entering consumer channels.

Food Preparation

Almost all cases of food poisoning resulting from microbial contamination of poultry can be prevented by proper preparation of the food. But this fact should not mitigate the responsibilities to protect public health delegated by the Congress to the Secretary of Agriculture. The committee endorses substantial efforts to improve food safety during food preparation, but does not believe that consumers can or should bear the sole responsibility for the microbial safety of the poultry they consume.

FSIS recognizes its responsibility to facilitate consumer understanding of proper food preparation. The committee did not review the agency's efforts to meet this responsibility, but it nonetheless urges USDA to obtain professional advice about the direction and purpose of its educational programs. Education is not a form of public relations, nor should it be regarded as a substitute for other actions. A successful program must almost certainly be multitargeted, reinforced by the mass media on a continuing basis, and formally evaluated periodically to be sure it is having the intended effects.

OVERALL EVALUATION

In the current FSIS inspection programs, considerable resources are devoted to some of the critical control points in the production system, but these activities have not been designed with an eye toward their evaluation and hence are not demonstrably effective. It also shows that because of the very nature of the poultry industry, it is less vulnerable to some risks than to others and that several control points are theoretically controlled by federal agencies other than those responsible for ensuring the safety of poultry products. In sum, resources are not always allocated to the right points and the resources that are properly directed are not achieving measured results. Major changes are required in the poultry inspection system if public health is to be protected and if the investment of resources is to have maximum effect.

REFERENCES

Anonymous. 1986. Streamline Inspection System (SIS). Fed. Vet. 43:3-4.

Blankenship, L. C., D. A. Shackelford, N. A. Cox, D. Burdick, J. S. Bailey, and J. E. Thomson. 1985. Survival of salmonellae as a function of poultry feed processing conditions. Pp. 211-220 in G. H. Snoyenbos, ed. Proceedings of the International Symposium on Salmonella held in New Orleans, Louisiana, July 19-20, 1984. American Association of Arian Pathologists , Kennett Square, Pa.

Bryan, F. L. 1978. Factors that contribute to outbreaks of foodborne disease. J. Food Protect. 41:816-827.

Bryan, F. L. 1980. Foodborne diseases in the United States associated with meat and poultry. J. Food Protect. 43:140-150.

CFR (Code of Federal Regulations). 1986a. Title 9, Animals and Animal Products; Section 381.19, Application for inspection; required facilities. U.S. Government Printing Office, Washington, D.C.

CFR (Code of Federal Regulations). 1986b. Title 21, Food and Drugs; Section 101.9, Nutrition labeling of food. U.S. Government Printing Office, Washington, D.C.

Cover, M. S., J. T. Gary, Jr., and S. F. Binder. 1985. Reduction of standard plate counts, total coliform counts and Salmonella by pelletizing animal feeds. Pp. 221-231 in G. H. Snoyenbos, ed. Proceedings of the International Symposium on Salmonella held in New Orleans, Louisiana, July 19-20, 1984. American Association of Arian Pathologists, Kennett Square, Pa.

Crittenden, L. B. 1979. The epidemiology of arian lymphoid leukosis. Cancer Res. 36:570-573.

Cruickshank, J. G., S. I. Egglestone, A. H. L. Gawler, and D. G. Lanning. 1982. Campylobacter jejuni and the broiler chicken process. Pp. 263-266 in the Proceedings of an International Workshop on Campylobacter, Epidemiology, Pathogenesis, and Biochemistry held at the University of Reading, England, March 24-26, 1981. MTP Press, Lancaster, United Kingdom.

Fenner, F., B. R. McAuslan, C. A. Mims, J. Sambrook, and D. O. White. 1974. Vital oncogenesis: RNA viruses. Pp. 508-542 in The Biology of Animal Viruses, 2nd ed. Academic Press, New York.

Green, S. S., A. B. Moran, R. W. Johnston, P. Uhler, and J. Chiu. 1982. The incidence of Salmonella species and serotypes in young whole chicken carcasses in 1979 as compared with 1967. Poult. Sci. 61:288-293.

Harris, N. V., N. S. Weiss, and C. M. Nolan. 1986. The role of poultry and meats in the etiology of Campylobacter jejuni/coli enteritis. Am. J. Public Health 76:407-411.

Holmberg, S. D., J. G. Wells, and M. L. Cohen. 1984. Animal-to-man transmission of antimicrobial-resistant Salmonella: Investigations of U.S. outbreaks, 1971-1983. Science 225:833-835.

Karel, M., and N. D. Heidelbaugh. 1975. Effects of packaging on nutrients. Pp. 412-462 in R. S. Harris and E. Karmas, eds. Nutritional Evaluation of Food Processing, 2nd ed. AVI Publishing, Westport, Conn.

Libby, J. A. 1975. Meat Hygiene, 4th ed. Lea & Febiger, Philadelphia. 658 pp.

NRC (National Research Council). 1979. Antibiotics in Animal Feeds. Report of the Committee on Animal Health and Committee on Animal Nutrition, Board on Agriculture and Renewable Resources. National Academy of Sciences, Washington, D.C. 53 pp.

NRC (National Research Council). 1980. The Effects on Human Health of Subtherapeutic Use of Antimicrobials in Animal Feeds. Report of the Committee to Study the Human Health Effects of Subtherapeutic Antibiotic Use in Animal Feeds, Division of Medical Sciences. National Academy of Sciences, Washington, D.C. 376 pp.

NRC (National Research Council). 1985. Meat and Poultry Inspection: The Scientific Basis of the Nation's Program. Report of the Committee on the Scientific Basis of the Nation's Meat and Poultry Inspection Program, Food and Nutrition Board. National Academy Press, Washington, D.C. 209 pp.

Sacharow, S. 1979. Packaging Regulations. AVI Publishing, Westport, Conn. 207 pp.

Settepani, J. A. 1984. The hazard of using chloramphenicol in food animals. J. Am. Vet. Med. Assoc. 184:930-931.

Shapcott, R. 1985. Practical aspects of Salmonella control: Progress report on a programme in a large broiler integration. Pp. 109-114 in G. H. Snoyenbos, ed. Proceedings of the International Symposium on Salmonella held in New Orleans, Louisiana, July 19-20, 1984. American Association of Arian Pathologists, Kennett Square, Pa.

USDA (U.S. Department of Agriculture). 1980. Report on the PCB Incident in the Western United States. Food Safety and Quality Service, U.S. Department of Agriculture, Washington, D.C. 122 pp.

USDA (U.S. Department of Agriculture). 1983a. Preoperational Sanitation Inspection in Poultry Slaughter Plants. MPI Bulletin 83-13, issued March 2, 1983. Meat and Poultry Inspection Operations, Food Safety and Inspection Service, U.S. Department of Agriculture, Washington, D.C. 9 pp.

USDA (U.S. Department of Agriculture). 1983b. Prevention—A new direction in reducing the risk of chemical residues in meat and poultry. Pp. 21-23 in Food Safety and Inspection Service Program Plan: Fiscal Year 1984. Food Safety and Inspection Service, U.S. Department of Agriculture, Washington, D.C.

USDA (U.S. Department of Agriculture). 1983c. Protection and Productivity: The Strategy for Meat and Poultry Inspection in the 1980's. Food Safety and Inspection Service, U.S. Department of Agriculture, Washington, D.C. 40 pp.

USDA (U.S. Department of Agriculture). 1984. Compound Evaluation and Analytical Capability. Science Program, Food Safety and Inspection Service, U.S. Department of Agriculture, Washington, D.C. [86 pp.]

USDA (U.S. Department of Agriculture). 1985a. Compound Evaluation and Analytical Capability: Annual Residue Plan. Science Program, Food Safety and Inspection Service, U.S. Department of Agriculture, Washington, D.C. [125 pp.]

USDA (U.S. Department of Agriculture). 1985b. Statistical Summary: Federal Meat and Poultry Inspection for Fiscal Year 1984. FSIS-14. Food Safety and Inspection Service, U.S. Department of Agriculture, Washington, D.C. 39 pp.

Williams, J. E. 1981. Salmonellas in poultry feed—a worldwide review. Parts I and II. World's Poult. Sci. J. 37:6-25.

Chapter 7

Conclusions and Recommendations

CONCLUSIONS

The Role of Risk Assessment

Risk assessment is a specialized and systematic means for organizing and presenting information about various types of health hazards, including those associated with the consumption of broiler chickens. Because it requires explicit, consistent, and logical treatment of data and their associated uncertainties, and consideration of current scientific knowledge, risk assessment is one of the most valuable tools available to serve regulatory agencies. Therefore, FSIS should begin a continuing program of more formalized applications of risk assessment based on a refined risk model, such as that proposed by the committee in Chapter 3, to analyze specific risks associated with poultry and to evaluate alternative strategies for managing these risks.

The data necessary to provide accurate quantitative risk assessments are not always available and vary greatly among the types of hazards presented by broiler chickens. Thus in many instances, particularly in connection with microbiological hazards, only qualitative assessments can now be done. The consistent use of the conceptual framework and model for all assessments ensures that current information is being used in the most effective possible way to guide risk management.

Although gaps in knowledge and lack of data limit the extent to which quantitative risk assessment can now be done, FSIS should consider the use of more formalized, and ultimately quantitative, risk assessment to serve as a foundation for important decisions involving issues of human health. Quantification is needed to clarify the magnitude of the various sources of human health risks and to provide a more defensible logic for decision making. Qualitative reasoning, even qualitative reasoning made more systematic by the use of a risk model, is often too vague and prone to error to serve as a satisfactory basis for definitive decisions bearing on human health. However, this reasoning does not necessarily lead to the conclusion that FSIS needs a highly detailed, comprehensive risk-assessment system to support its decision making. Some initial efforts to quantify the framework chosen should reveal whether further quantitation will be cost effective and the extent to which risk assessment, in general, will be useful.

Risk assessment is not the only component of a regulatory program. Although protection of the public from significant health risks is the ultimate goal of any FSIS program, the types and range of risk-management options are influenced by legal, regulatory, and historical precedents that cannot be ignored by decision makers. The committee has dealt only with the ways in which risk assessment can assume a more prominent role in the decisions made by FSIS in the absence of such constraints.

The Risk Model

The committee believes that the conceptual framework and risk model developed in Chapter 3 and examples of their application in assessing the risks presented by microbial contamination and chemical residues (Chapters 4 and 5) should serve as a guide in future FSIS data-gathering and risk-assessment activities. In Chapter 6, the committee used this analytical approach to identify risk-management options and to evaluate FSIS programs and activities. In so doing, it learned much about the adequacy of current FSIS programs. The recommendations set forth below are based on this evaluation.

Current FSIS Programs

The committee's use of the risk model in earlier chapters of this report was designed not only to illustrate how risk assessment can be used to evaluate current programs and to guide the development of future ones but also to answer the following question: Are current FSIS inspection techniques reasonably related to the level of public health risk associated with various components of the broiler chicken risk model?

By applying the risk model developed in Chapter 3, the committee observed that the traditional postmortem inspection system cannot deal with several sources of risk at certain points in production and distribution due to limitations of FSIS authority. Among these are the assignment of acceptable daily intake (ADI) or other levels of tolerable intake for chemical residues, monitoring of poultry feed and drinking water to prevent contamination of the products, and education of the consumer regarding safe poultry preparation practices. Effective risk-management programs must include a range of activities that fall outside traditional postmortem inspection. Some of the committee's recommendations derive from this conclusion.

Microbial Hazards. As stated in Chapter 3, the committee believes that the present system of inspection provides little opportunity to detect or control the most significant health risks associated with broiler chickens. Although information is not sufficient for the committee to conclude that the FSIS inspection program has no public health benefits, the weight of the evidence does suggest that the current program can not provide effective protection against the risks presented by microbial agents that are pathogenic to humans. The committee believes that alternative and potentially less costly strategies, which are described below, may provide greater benefits to public health. An integral component of these strategies is the use of a statistically based sampling plan, rather than the traditional approach of 100% inspection. Some details of a possible approach are described in the recommendations presented below under Sampling Procedures.

Current inspection procedures do not significantly reduce contamination of broilers by microorganisms that are pathogenic to humans, nor were they designed to do so. Even if they were to be responsible for small reductions in contamination levels, however, there are further opportunities for increasing or decreasing microbial contamination after the products leave FSIS control. For example, cross-contamination can occur during distribution and food preparation; proper cooking can effectively eliminate microbial risks. These factors affect both Salmonella and Campylobacter, which are among the major causes of food-borne morbidity among humans in the United States.

Since the current system of postmortem poultry inspection is not an effective device for managing this public health problem, several types of corrective action should be taken. Furthermore, other microbial risks need to be investigated with greater vigor, and additional data should be sought so that the magnitude of the public risk associated with microbial contaminants can be assessed more accurately. These constitute the committee's central conclusions regarding FSIS inspection programs. The recommendations presented below derive from them.

Chemical Hazards. Unlike microbial risks, the relationship between chemical contamination levels in poultry at the slaughterhouse and on the dinner plate is much better understood. In this case, critical factors and uncertainties in the risk model concern the nature, likelihood, and level of chemical residues and the health effects produced by the ingestion of those residues. The problem is therefore analogous to other chemical risk management problems, which have been addressed effectively through an approach based on the establishment of maximum permissible concentrations.

It seems clear, however, that there has been insufficient investigation of the possible extent of the problem of chemical residues in poultry. A comprehensive analysis of the potential risk of chemical residues in poultry was therefore not possible, but in examining the limited data available the committee found no evidence that such residues pose a sigificant threat to public health. The committee's recommendations in this area are designed to encourage systematic investigation of the problem and to increase the efficiency of current inspection efforts.

Current monitoring programs are designed primarily to detect a given frequency of tolerance violations. This objective may not be compatible with public health protection—the principal goal of FSIS inspection. It does not, for example, take into account the fact that the potential public health risks posed by chemical residues vary considerably. Several recommendations concern the means to reorient current monitoring programs.

In general, it appears that FSIS programs are directed more toward detecting of macroscopic problems rather than toward investigating the origins of health hazards and finding ways to solve them. The detection of microbial and chemical contaminants as part of a quality assurance program designed to assist in revealing their sources would be a commendable addition to current efforts. The general tone of all recommendations derives from these observations.

RECOMMENDATIONS

General

- Risk assessment based on the conceptual framework and a risk model such as that provided in Chapter 3 should be used to guide FSIS risk-management programs. Examples of how these may be applied to assessments of microbiological and chemical hazards and to program evaluation are given in Chapters 4, 5, and 6.
- Current poultry inspection programs are primarily concerned with detecting diseased and damaged poultry so that very few of the problems detected by this system are threats to public health. Because federal funding of the inspection program is intended to protect public health, it seems clear that such funds should be expended in direct proportion to the magnitude of the public health risks. Qualitative risk assessments should be used to determine where the major risks occur, how they might be controlled, and consequently to which aspects of the inspection program funds should be diverted. When needed, quantitative risk assessments may be required to elucidate complex health risks.
- Rather than focusing on one procedure, such as bird-by-bird inspection, as the primary component of an inspection process, FSIS should direct its efforts toward the establishment of a comprehensive quality assurance program. Such a program would consist of several components, one of which might be organoleptic inspection.

- An important component of any quality assurance program is a statistically based random sampling protocol. The committee recommends that FSIS establish such a sampling program as part of any future modifications of its inspection system.
- Emphasis should be shifted from detection to prevention of problems at the earliest feasible stage in production to increase the effectiveness of poultry risk-management activities.
- In the areas of risk management outside the purview of FSIS, the agency should attempt to maintain a close liaison with responsible agencies.

Microbiological Contaminants

- FSIS should use the tools of risk assessment to establish priorities for a risk-management program to protect consumers from microbiological hazards using the tools of risk assessment. Relevant activities are:

Identify and evaluate potentially pathogenic microorganisms found on poultry products.

Determine the potential for exposure to an infectious dose of pathogens derived from contaminated poultry products.

Evaluate the potential public health impact of failure to control each of the identified microbial hazards.

- FSIS should identify and monitor the critical control points of the poultry system at which microorganisms pathogenic to humans are introduced. This will assist industry in identifying production practices that result in exposure of consumers to poultry-borne pathogens.
- Because fecal contamination is a primary source of the microbial load on broiler carcasses, FSIS should identify and monitor critical control points within dressing procedures to prevent soilage of carcasses by intestinal contents and carcass-to-carcass contamination.
- In describing the risk model (Chapter 3), the committee identified a variety of points in the slaughtering process where operations involving machinery have the potential to influence contamination levels. Application of this risk model to microbial risks in Chapter 4 led to the conclusion that several of these operations had a critical bearing on the levels of _Salmonella_ on carcasses. Hence, greater emphasis should be given to the operation, maintenance, and improvement of machinery (e.g., pluckers and chillers) to reduce the likelihood of microbial contamination in slaughterhouses.
- FSIS should begin to lay the groundwork for a shift from the organoleptic inspection of each broiler chicken to a program that is more likely to have a substantial impact on human

health and disease. Further development of quantitative health risk assessment will be an essential tool in this change.

- Educational programs for people who handle raw broilers in slaughterhouses, at retail, and during food preparation in the home and in commercial establishments should be established or intensified to alert them of the potential risks and to instruct them in proper food handling practices. As part of this effort, all poultry products inspected by FSIS should be labeled at retail to inform consumers about the optimal ways to protect themselves from microbial hazards.
- Community-based surveillance of pathogens on poultry products and of food-borne disease incidence in humans should be intensified to measure the success of programs undertaken to reduce the prevalence of human pathogens on market-ready poultry and the direct impact of program activities on the public's health.
- FSIS should ensure that it can achieve the above objectives either by its own activities or through agreements with other agencies having appropriate authority and expertise.

Chemical Residues

- To protect consumers from chemical residues in poultry products, FSIS should adopt a risk-management program that includes the following activities (some of which would require close coordination or agreements with other agencies):

  Identify hazardous substances that could appear as residues in poultry products.

  Establish ADIs or other levels of tolerable daily intake of such substances by humans.

  Establish tolerances for residue levels in edible poultry products and institute enforcement programs to ensure that those levels are not exceeded.

  Establish levels of intake for poultry through diet, drinking water, or other sources to ensure that tolerances in poultry products are not exceeded.

  Establish control programs to ensure that poultry feed, drinking water, or other sources of chemical residues do not contain chemicals of concern at levels exceeding those identified in the preceding activity.

  Establish procedures that provide for efficient removal of contaminated poultry products from commerce.

  Identify priorities for each activity described above using the concepts and tools of risk assessment.

- FSIS should categorize chemicals according to source, as described in Chapter 5, to assist in the identification of risk-management responsibilities and objectives.
- FSIS should ensure that it has in place programs to carry out all activities not clearly assigned to FDA (tolerance setting for additives and drug residues), to EPA (tolerance setting for pesticides), or to other agencies.
- In USDA research programs, emphasis should be given to accidental chemical contaminants, environmental contaminants, and chemicals formed during processing, storage, and heating of poultry products. The current Exploratory Testing Program should be expanded to include research on the following essential topics: the toxic properties of chemical agents (to assist in setting acceptable intake levels), levels in poultry products, and methods of chemical analysis.
- In cooperation with FDA and EPA, FSIS should learn the extent to which the existing data on chemicals intentionally administered or applied to poultry or poultry feed are adequate to support current tolerance levels.
- A prevention program to monitor poultry feed and drinking water should be seriously considered as the first line of defense against residues in poultry products. Such programs could be undertaken using procedures recommended by FSIS. Close cooperation with FDA may be necessary to achieve this objective. Data necessary to implement such a program (i.e., data on maximum acceptable feed and water levels) should already be available for intentionally used substances. Additional research is necessary to establish feed and drinking water limits for environmental chemicals and accidental contaminants.
- The committee recommends that priorities for monitoring feed, water, and poultry products and the intensity of the monitoring efforts be directly related to the relative magnitudes of risk posed by candidate substances should they escape detection and enter the marketplace. Priorities for research should be assigned in the same way. A methodology for assessing relative risks is presented in Chapter 5 (Activity 8).
- FSIS should periodically assess the public health risks of chemical residues in poultry products, using data collected from its residue monitoring program together with data on toxicity. Monitoring and enforcement should be increased or decreased, according to the results of these assessments.

Sampling Procedures

The quality and safety of poultry products are linked closely to the occurrence of chemical and microbiological contaminants that may originate from a variety of sources. To ensure the safety of retail products, contaminants must be minimized. This is most effectively accomplished by detecting them as early as possible in the poultry system and preventing their introduction by contolling the source, for example, by sampling and testing the water and feed of growing chickens. However, preinspection components of the poultry system are outside FSIS jurisdiction. Therefore, any sampling program adopted by FSIS incorporating, for example, an effort to monitor microbial counts during slaughter should be complemented by collaborative efforts with FDA and EPA to monitor the microbial load of feed that might have been contaminated by rodents or that might contain improperly sterilized animal by-products. One possible scheme for monitoring chickens during slaughter is presented below using the format of a three-stage sampling scheme.

The committee recommends that FSIS develop and maintain close liaison with programs that monitor the acceptability of feed and water supplied to growing chickens and substantially expand its own sampling program to assess the quality of poultry products and, most importantly, the human health hazards of freshly slaughtered birds. To accomplish this, FSIS should consider the following three-stage sampling scheme developed by the committee.

In the first stage, a random number generator (functioning independently from plant quality control programs), a counter, and a signal attached to the line could flag birds with a probability (p) of removal from the line and mark them for detailed inspection. The sampling fraction R might be set at 1/500 or 1/5,000 (or higher or lower), depending on plant history, past performance of the grower, and other factors. Plant inspection staff should have a role only in determining how many birds are chosen, not which birds are chosen. Sampled birds would be marked to identify flock and time of inspection, for example, and hung on a rack for organoleptic examination in groups (perhaps by flocks) in a manner substantially more detailed than at present. This sample inspection would of course not preclude additional inspection of the present type or other types that might be deemed appropriate by the inspector in charge; it provides a minimum for FSIS involvement, not a maximum. This first-stage inspection would have several purposes:

- to maintain awareness of the quality of the product at this stage, including detection of gross disease and malfunctioning equipment;
- to ensure that FSIS can fulfill its statutory mandate;
- to provide direction for further studies, especially laboratory studies of microbial and chemical hazards;
- to exert pressure on poultry processors to apply inspection procedures that conform to acceptable standards; and
- to provide data that could serve as a basis for further modification of the sampling system, e.g., in the size of the samples, in inspection techniques, and in objectives.

The committee recognizes the appearance of a disjunction between earlier statements that organoleptic inspection has no demonstrated health value and this recommendation to continue organoleptic inspection of a small percentage of slaughtered birds. There is no contradiction, however, since the recommended inspection of the sample is not intended to detect and condemn defective birds individually but, rather, to provide a continuing source of information about how the poultry industry responds to the shift from treatment to prevention of problems, to ensure that plant inspection does not deteriorate to the extent that new health hazards are presented, and to maintain awareness of changes in a flock's condition or in equipment performance that may have health implications. It may in time become apparent that this phase of sampling can be omitted under some conditions, for example, when a producer has a very strong quality control program of its own and a long history of minimal problems in the samples, but the committee does not recommend the complete omission of this step under existing conditions.

In the second stage of sampling, most birds selected in the first stage would be returned to the line, but a random subsample would be retained for still more detailed study, including simple laboratory studies for microbial load and chemical residues at the plant. The sample must again be strictly random, perhaps by rack location (randomized anew each time). Sampling fractions might be anywhere from 1/20 to 1/500, depending again on the past record of the supplier and the past performance of the plant. The purpose of this stage is surveillance for specific, direct microbial and chemical risks to health to ensure a timely response and correction as needed. Flocks may be fully processed and shipped before any of the test results are available, but the primary goal of this sampling would have been met, that is, to develop a needed information base, not now available, on health hazards as they appear at this very critical point in the process. Recall of birds or parts found to have very serious problems might be feasible. Thus, an effort should be made to find and implement rapid testing procedures that will make it possible to remove contaminated birds before they reach the retail market.

In the third stage, a further random subsample of the second stage would be frozen or otherwise preserved and sent to a central laboratory for studies not feasible at the plant. This would in essence continue and expand the present scope of NRP sampling, and methods and sampling fractions should be adjusted to both the information need and the work load that NRP can accommodate. The purpose and justification would be similar to those supporting present NRP activities. Chemical testing would probably dominate this stage, but the committee believes that opportunities for further microbial testing should be examined by FSIS. This subsample should be subjected to morphologic and etiologic diagnoses to help build a data base against which future program activities can be measured.

The committee also recommends that the present size and composition of the NRP sample be reexamined in light of data needs and resource allocations within the overall inspection program proposed by the committee. With the present random sampling of 300 chickens per year, some plants and some large producers may not be sampled for years at a stretch and even major problems. that are localized in space or time (accidents) may be overlooked and thus not resolved in a timely fashion. In short, the stated goal of a 95% probability of finding a chemical contaminant present in 1% of birds slaughtered during a single year may not be sufficiently protective of the public health to meet current expectations. However, it would be unrealistic to sample the entire U.S. population of chickens as if they are a homogeneous group. The sample size required would be unmanageably large. Instead, FSIS should develop an appropriate sampling structure based, for example, on homogeneous and useful units like rearing groups, or random lots of birds characterized by some common feature such as their point of origin. (Recommendations for matching sampling rate to relative risks are presented above under Chemical Residues.)

Sampling of feed, water, and processed products is likely to be less complex than sampling of birds on the line, and FSIS already has programs in place or models to follow. The committee emphasizes, however, that expert technical support should be provided to ensure that sampling plans meet program goals in a technically sound and cost-effective manner.